D0886966

More than Herbs
and Acupuncture

More than Herbs and Acupuncture

E. GREY DIMOND, M.D.

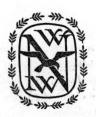

W · W · NORTON & COMPANY · INC·

New York

FIRST EDITION

This book was typeset in Linotype Janson. Composition, printing, and binding were done by the Vail-Ballou Press, Inc.

Library of Congress Cataloging in Publication Data
Dimond, Edmunds Grey, 1918–
    More than herbs and acupuncture.
    1. Medicine—China. 2. Medicine, Chinese.
3. China—Description and travel—1949– I. Title.
[DNLM: 1. Acupuncture. 2. Medicine—China.
3. Public health—China. WB50 JC6 D5m]
R601.D55 1975   610′951   74–11166

ISBN 0-393-06400-X

1 2 3 4 5 6 7 8 9 0

CONTENTS

Appendices   *197*

More than Herbs
and Acupuncture

Chapter One

TO CHINA VIA DUBLIN,
NEW HAMPSHIRE

I met Edgar Snow in Dublin, New Hampshire, in 1965. He was one of a group of fifty who had gathered there at the urging of Grenville Clark to explore the possibilities of a workable form of international understanding, not based on military action, that would reduce the risks to mankind in the absence of such an understanding.*

The participants, including Paul Dudley White, Norman Cousins, Kingman Brewster, Gerard Piel, Harlow Shapley, James P. Warburg, Erwin N. Griswold, John Jessup, and others, were stimulating, but the man who brought real excitement to the gathering was the expatriate American author, Edgar Snow.

Snow was neither a Communist nor a Communist sympathizer. He was an extremely accurate reporter, who, by hard work and luck, had achieved a reporter's ultimate dream and had scooped the world with his original interviews with Mao and his documentary book, *Red Star over China*, in 1939.

Parenthetically, anyone today wanting to understand the People's Republic of China should begin by reading Snow's *Red Star*. There is no other place to begin, in any language, including Chinese.

After the Dublin meeting, Snow and I kept in contact. I was at his home in Nyon, Switzerland, in April, 1969, and in June, 1970, and we kept letters going back and forth.

In the fall of 1970, Snow was in China, and the clear message that the Chinese would accept a visit by the American President was given directly to Snow by Mao Tse-tung. The interview was

* This meeting resulted in the Second Dublin Conference Statement. See Appendix A.

widely circulated in China and was the first signal to the Chinese people that change of attitude toward Americans was developing.

The significance of this interview was enhanced when Mao Tse-tung invited Snow to his side on the reviewing wall of the Tien en Men Gate during the October First celebration. This smiling photograph of the two with the full identification "Edgar Snow, American friend" was circulated widely in China. Snow's article and the photograph also appeared in *Life* magazine in the United States and encouraged President Nixon and Dr. Henry Kissinger in their plan to visit Peking, which marked the end of the United States' Taiwan policy.

During Snow's 1970 visit, he saw a great deal of China's new health care program, developed subsequent to the Cultural Revolution of 1966. This was facilitated by his long friendship with the American-born physician, George Hatem, now a Chinese citizen, Dr. Ma Hai-teh. Although Dr. Ma Hai-teh was able to give Snow accurate information on much of China's health care policy, he spoke with special authority on the successful elimination of venereal disease and prostitution. From another old friend, Dr. Lin Ch'iao-chih, chief of obstetrics and gynecology at a primary hospital in Peking, Snow got a firsthand account of China's massive educational program in family planning and birth control. Snow followed the health care system out to the vast commune developments and saw the Chinese version of the physician's assistant, the barefoot doctor. All of this he described in three articles that appeared in the *New Republic* in early 1971.

There was one area of medicine that Snow saw and reported upon but simply did not feel competent to judge. This was the use of acupuncture as anesthesia for major surgery. He told me of his impression and his concern. He had seen major operations, including brain and chest surgery, in which, seemingly, the anesthesia resulted from the twirling of needles at distant points. For example, the manipulation of one needle in the forearm had been the only anesthetic for a major chest incision and lung removal. Could this be true? Was this possible? Was this hypnosis? Was the result possible only in China and under the persuasion of Mao Tse-tung Thought?

Snow urged me to make the trip to China and see if, from a physician's viewpoint, I could find evidence that this was a valid procedure. I told him that I would go, of course, if a visa was offered, look as critically as I could, and give him an opinion, but I pointed out that the issue was one in which one's judgment would be seriously doubted by the American medical profession.

From what Snow told me, it was evident that the drama and publicity attending acupuncture anesthesia would be great. The picture of a smiling, talking, eating and drinking patient undergoing surgery free of pain and without medicated anesthesia was clearly high theater. The American medical witness who first went, saw, and reported to his colleagues would need to write in a matter-of-fact tone and straightforward style, free of any suggestion of personal gain or involvement. No matter how low-keyed, such a report in the American medical literature was bound to be overinterpreted and exaggerated beyond the author's intent.

But the whole story of the health care program in China needed to be understood, not acupuncture anesthesia alone. The role of the barefoot doctor, of herbs, of massive public health measures, of changes in medical education, were all areas needing an accurate medical analysis. Therefore, when Snow urged me to take on the task of opening the medical relationships between our countries and reporting on medicine in China, I suggested that Paul Dudley White should go with me. My reason for this was twofold. First, Paul White was one of our most respected senior medical figures, and my opinions about China, backed by his, would have a degree of authenticity that would make the skeptic hesitate before voicing criticism. Secondly, and of equal merit, Dr. White had tried for years to include China in his serious efforts in world friendship. Snow agreed with this line of logic, and added that my wife, Mary Clark Dimond, the daughter of Grenville Clark, should also be invited. Thus the original relationships begun in Dublin, New Hampshire, led to these plans in the spring of 1971. Snow conveyed our plan directly to Chou En-lai and formally recommended me to him.

My previous international experiences included:

1956 • Fulbright Professor to the Netherlands
1956 • Paul White Traveling Scholarship to India, Thailand, Philippines, Taiwan, and Japan
1959 • Visiting professor, Institute of Cardiology, London
1962 • Visiting professor, Philippines and Taiwan, on behalf of the U.S. State Department
1963 • Visiting professor, Colombia and Chile, on behalf of the U.S. State Department
1964 • Visiting professor, Nigeria and Sudan, on behalf of the U.S. State Department
1965 • Visiting professor, Czechoslovakia, Ceylon, Indonesia, and Vietnam, on behalf of the U.S. State Department

Fellows and students from these countries had been in my laboratory. My main intent was always the teaching of cardiology, but my learning about the rest of the world was an associated dividend. Changes in world power were occurring without most Americans knowing, or perhaps caring. The interesting possibility of a world in which China would have an important, if not dominant, influence is a new idea for Western man.

Specifically, a remarkable race of man, the Chinese, is about to enter for the first time the full world scene. The largest race, the oldest culture, impressively organized, under a disciplined, cohesive system, is about to become an influence, a force—economically, militarily, and morally. And Western man has no antecedent experience to prepare him for this historical event.

Had a godless regime, with the elimination of the energetic guidance of the well-meaning Christian efforts of the United States, England, France, Germany, Russia, Italy, Spain, in a brief twenty-two years cleaned up an entire collection of problems? Were the people happy? If so, how could this be?

A long-time scholar of Chinese history, John King Fairbank, defined the West's dilemma: "The Chinese Communist rise to power in 1949 called into question our own view of ourselves and our place in the world process. Insofar as the missionary conversion and the general uplift of the Chinese people had expressed our conviction that we lead the march of human progress, our self-confidence was dealt a grievous blow. One-fourth of mankind in China spurned not only Christianity, but also the supremacy of law, the ideals of individualism, the multi-party election process, civil liberties, and the self-determination of peoples, indeed our entire political order and its concepts of freedom and security through due process. We felt our basic value directly menaced. One consolation in this crisis, therefore, was to think that the new Chinese Communist dictatorship did not represent the interests of a large enough proportion of the Chinese people, that it maintained itself only by force and manipulation, that, in fact, it was too evil to last, and in any case must be opposed as a matter of principle and duty."

Edgar Snow was the only American citizen who had been able to maintain contact with Mao Tse-tung and Chou En-lai. He had been in China in 1960 and 1965 and he himself had been surprised and taken aback by the ferocity of the Cultural Revolution of 1966 and the turning out of Liu Shao-ch'i. After his five and a half months there in the winter of 1970 and 1971, he summarized his observations in part in the three articles in the *New Republic* and made it clear in his title, "Talks with Chou En-lai: The Open Door," that China was ready for further advances from the United States.

Chapter Two

A BRIEFING BY EDGAR SNOW

PRESIDENT NIXON had begun efforts early in his first term to open conversations with China. Various probes were made, and de Gaulle's help was directly requested, but the absolute lack of interchange made beginning conversations difficult.

On April 14, 1971, the U.S. table tennis team, which had been in Japan, was suddenly in Peking. Prior to that, two American biologists had entered China from North Vietnam. They were Ethan R. Signer from the Massachusetts Institute of Technology and Arthur W. Galston of Yale.

In July, Dr. Henry Kissinger's arrival in Peking was not only a world surprise but so crushing a blow to the reporter's instinct of James Reston of the New York *Times,* that the Reston appendix rebelled and required Peking surgery. Mr. Reston had made almost a triumphal entry as one of the first reporters (not counting Snow) to obtain a visa. After arriving in China, he was encouraged to take a forty-hour train trip from Canton to Peking, learning only later that the real reason for the slow journey was the need to tuck him away quietly on the train until Dr. Kissinger completed his visit. One of the best bits of good humor was Mr. Reston's paragraph of July 25, 1971, from Peking: "Without a single shred of supporting medical evidence, I can trace my attack of acute appendicitis to Henry A. Kissinger of the White House staff. He arrived in China on July 9th. My wife and I arrived in south China the day before, just in time.

"But when we reached Canton, we were told by our official guide that there had been a change in our plans. We were to remain in the Canton area for two days and proceed by rail to Peking on the evening of the 10th, arriving in the capital on the morning of the 12th. . . .

"Three days later, at precisely 10:30 A.M., while I was describing to several Foreign Ministry officials . . . the unquestionable advantages of my interviewing Chairman Mao Tse-tung, Premier Chou, and every other prominent official I could think of, Chen Chu, the head of the Ministry's information service, interrupted to say that he had 'a little news item.' Mr. Kissinger had been in Peking from July 9 to July 11, he said, and it was now being announced here and in the United States that President Nixon would visit Peking before May, 1972.

"At that precise moment, or so it seems now, the first stab of pain went through my groin. By evening I had a temperature of 103, and in my delirium I could see Mr. Kissinger floating across my bedroom ceiling and grinning at me out of the corner of a hooded rickshaw."

After my conversations with Snow in the early springtime of 1971, I followed the reports of visits by Americans with enthusiasm. However, April, May, June, and July passed with absolutely no information. August came and still no news. Finally, on August 22, I received a letter from Snow which said he thought a visit in 1971 was unlikely and that I should not expect an invitation for another year. This seemed definite and final.

Forty-eight hours later, the long-distance operator rang me in Kansas City and said I had a call from Geneva, Switzerland. It was Edgar, and he came quickly to the point. "Did you get my letter? Disregard it! The Chinese have invited you to come for three months to take a thorough look at medicine. They want you there by September 15."

It is astonishing how excited one can become over what is essentially a simple act. It is also amazing how complicated life can be in our age of rapid communication and movement. In the sixteen days before our date of entry from Hong Kong, we opened a new medical school in Kansas City, flew to Ottawa, Canada, to get our visas from the Chinese Embassy, flew to Helsinki, Finland, for a medical seminar on coronary disease, flew to Switzerland to visit the Snows, flew to Hong Kong to rendezvous with Paul and Ina White.

The visit to see the Snows in Nyon was a special opportunity which, in a sense, was an intensive course on modern China. Edgar and his wife, Lois Wheeler Snow, had completed their own

five-month trip to China in early 1971, and both were heavily
involved in writing—not only articles, but each was at work on
the manuscript of a book. This briefing by Edgar and Lois was a
remarkable advantage for Mary and me, and from this beginning
we were able to quickly establish contacts and friendships with
Edgar's friends in China. Among these especially were Ma Hai-
teh, Hans Müller, and Rewi Alley.

Edgar's writing was going slow. In China he had not felt
well at all times and on the way home had spent a few days in
the hospital in Hong Kong. Since returning to Nyon, he had
suffered from some nagging health problems and had tried several
forms of therapy. He was finding it difficult to place his material
with American publishers, and his spirits were a little low, but
the excitement associated with our going to China as a result of
his help buoyed the visit. On our last night in Nyon, Edgar
declared it a special occasion and produced a white ceramic con-
tainer with a vivid red label. This, he announced, was the great
Chinese white wine, Mao-tai, used for toasting special occasions.
He poured for the four of us minuscule amounts of perhaps
20 cc and gave a farewell, bon voyage toast.

Mao-tai is a drink to be respected. Twenty cc is plenty. It is
a colorless drink served straight without ice. It is made from grain
and has the reputed alcohol content of 80 percent, which means
it is 160 proof. Not only is it strong in alcohol content, but one
would have to be trained over a considerable period of time to
acquire a taste for Mao-tai. There is a special characteristic of
Mao-tai that can be best characterized as its "three-second effect."
In odor and flavor, it is immediately recognizable upon swallow-
ing as a strong drink but possible. Then, after a three-second
delay, there is an aftertaste which makes one rapidly reach for a
chaser, be it orangeade, beer, or water. This delayed taste must
take considerable practice to learn to appreciate. However, there
is a certain feeling of good fellowship that comes from a toast
offered with Mao-tai. Surely the toaster means well or he would
not expose himself to such a violent liquid.

Edgar reviewed with us Chinese history from the Boxer
Rebellion through the Cultural Revolution. Especially exciting
was his analysis of the Chinese leaders as he had known them for

thirty years. Equally useful was his explanation of terms that had appeared in the material I had read but that had not made clear logic to me. For example, I did not understand the slogan, "Struggle—Criticism—Transformation," which was evidently a fundamental mechanism of persuasion, Chinese style. What did it mean? Edgar explained that, in his mind, the phrase identified what was the essence of the difference between Russian Communism and Chinese Communism.

He pointed out that in Russia, as he had seen it, if one strayed from the Party line, the official response was punitive and that the constant threat of arrest, imprisonment, concentration camp, removal to Siberia, and even death had produced a style of citizenship in which there was a degree of real fear for one's safety.

Mao's technique has been one of carefully defining the Party line and then, through what in the West would be forceful group dynamics and encounter groups, giving the wayward, misguided, or obstructive citizen every chance to "reorient his thinking." The phrase "Struggle—Criticism—Transformation" was used to express this general tactic. Such interplay usually went on in the individual's place of work or school. Specific periods of time were set aside for working colleagues to sit down together and, one after the other, engage in self-criticism of one's own performance and cross-criticism throughout the group. All levels of employees met together. For example, in a hospital, the chief of a service, the nurses, the young house staff, the ward help, the janitor, and the in-residence representative of the Communist Party would meet, as much as a half day a week, to discuss thoroughly each other's performance—was one's job done well, was it done happily, was it done with a lack of self-interest, was it done without self-aggrandizement, was the individual performing as he should in a classless society, was he practicing and demonstrating the very best principles of Marxism, Leninism, and Maoism?

I interrupted Edgar to ask for a simple, functional statement of what these principles meant—Marxism, Leninism, and Maoism. Edgar said that we should come to that later, but first he wanted to finish his description of the methods used by Mao, which were essentially those of moral persuasion rather than those of a police state. Edgar cautioned me with the reminder that he was not ignoring the violence that had accompanied certain stages of the Communists' implementation of their policies.

Edgar pointed out that such repeated personal discussions with all of one's associates would solve many administrative problems in any part of the world, and, in fact, were a good basic principle of administration. Combining this with the national program, which steadily proclaimed that leaders must serve the people and not assume the airs of a bureaucracy and forget that the intent is a classless, socialized society, and, added to these talks, the presence of a Party representative . . . well, it was safe to assume that most points of contention would be solved.

What if such on-job group critiques still did not persuade the individual to be a better citizen? Did arrest follow?

Not at all. First, the Party member would recommend some intensive study of Mao's writings. Special classes were available to help the unreconstructed one through a considerable reading and group discussion program. The recalcitrant individual would usually find a way to understand how he had been wrong, and then, frequently, when next meeting with his colleagues, would criticize himself and identify his faults, and tell how he had come to see the light, how he had resolved the "contradiction," and how he would do better in the future. The period of struggle and criticism could be extremely volatile and even threatening to the target person in the degree of intimidation, humiliation, and harassment.*

"But," I asked, "what if the individual simply persevered in his attitude. For example, if a physician was careless about his records, would not complete his charts, was critical of the nurses, would not help in the outpatient clinic, and yet insisted that, as a physican, he was the senior member of the health team and was not going to tolerate having the staff criticize him. After all, he was in charge, had the major responsibility, and if he was not able to run things as he wanted to, he would quit."

Such a man was limited in what this threat could accomplish.

* The "struggle" is in the sense of verbal and psychic asault, not physical blows. This is a generally accurate statement; however, at the peak of the Cultural Revolution physical assault was reported.

Quitting was not the same as in the United States, where it meant he would try to get a new job elsewhere. In China, one cannot change his location and means of contributing to the people (working) at his discretion, but must have the approval of the Party.

Our stubborn doctor usually would not be transferred but would be recommended for a May 7 School for an indefinite period of time. May 7 Schools are available—hundreds of them—for the thousands of managers, leaders, doctors, teachers, intellectuals, and officials who need a periodic "touching up" of social awareness. These schools are named in recognition of Chairman Mao's directive of May 7, 1966, which said: "Going down to the countryside to do manual labor gives vast numbers of cadres [leaders] and excellent opportunity to study once again."

I interrupted to suggest that the Chairman certainly had some kindly phrases for clothing rather heavy-handed tactics. Edgar smiled and advised me to hold my analysis until I had been there. He continued: "When our wayward doctor receives his instructions to report to a specific May 7 School, he has no knowledge of how long he will remain there 'to be re-educated by the poor and lower-middle peasants.' It may be six months or several years."

His life in the May 7 School would not be medical but would be a mixture of planned study of the writings of Mao, Marx, Lenin, and Engels and intensive discussion groups analyzing how to apply this information to the problems of China and, equally, to the international political scene. Each day there would be physical labor, such as working in the fields, making bricks, and even helping to build his own living quarters. A May 7 School is not a reform school with guards and walls but is a reforming school with the objective, through persuasion, of making our physician able to talk and think of Marxist principles and of how to conduct himself as a model "serve the people" citizen. Our doctor would remain there until he was able to understand his errors and then, as with the majority of May 7 students, would return to his original job. A few students would decide to settle permanently "in the countryside." This last remark gave me a start, and I asked if he meant a concentration camp. Edgar's answer was to imply that the individual had moved his career from the city to a rural area, and that for a doctor this simply meant he was going to practice in a commune.

I could only say that this sounded considerably like a form of punishment, and in fact the whole procedure called "persuasion" gave me chills. Edgar agreed that there was a definite theme in the Chinese method which said to the citizens, "Here is what we expect of you; if you persist in obstruction, you will be criticized by your colleagues. If that does not influence you to do better, then you will have a thorough schooling at a May 7 School, away from your family, work, and home. If that does not influence you to do better, then you will be asked to work at a new task more in keeping with your level of 'social conscience,' and this often is in a remote rural area or in a newly settled frontier area. The door is always open for you to be rehabilitated and to return to your original work provided you have decided to become a model citizen of new China." Edgar and I agreed that this was strong interference with personal liberty, but then, said Edgar, how can you save a sinking ship or nation unless everyone works at the task? China had been a miserable, starving, pest-ridden, occupied land. To rebuild it left no room for dissent.

I broke in and said to Edgar that I did not understand what he meant by Marxist principles and I didn't understand what he meant by Mao-Tse-tung Thought. Edgar laughed, raised his thimble of Mao-tai, and said, "Here's to your China education! *Ganbei!* Come back after your trip and let's pick up the next lesson."

I retorted that the Mao technique of persuasion, although free of guns and chains, was one of saying, "You behave or else." Edgar laughed and suggested that perhaps the right expression was, "When eight hundred million people are on the brink of disaster, you behave or else."

The next lesson, of course, was canceled by Snow's overwhelming illness.

Chapter Three

DOWN THE MOUNTAIN WITH
PAUL DUDLEY WHITE

ON THE LONG FLIGHT from Geneva, I used the time to learn more about China and to prepare a list to submit to the Chinese Medical Association of things I wanted to accomplish.

In my notebook I made a list of facts and perhaps useful guides: Land mass of China is the same as continental U.S.A. Between 750 million and 850 million people, and no one knows exactly how many. Eighty percent of this entire population within 500 miles of the seacoast on the east. Eighty-five percent of the population actively farming. Immense cities I have never heard of, all larger than Cleveland, or Washington, or Dallas: Ch'ang-ch'un, Fu-shun, T'ai-yüan, Ch'eng-tu, Lü-ta. Or the province of Honan with 48 million, almost one-fourth of the United States' total population. How could we know so little about so many?

The sea of people involved became more significant as I tabulated the number of Chinese and began adding in a parallel column the population of other nations:

China	800,000,000	U.S.A.	209,200,000
		Ireland	3,000,000
		France	51,900,000
		Norway	4,000,000
		Denmark	5,000,000
		Belgium	9,800,000
		Austria	7,500,000
		Sweden	8,200,000
		Netherlands	13,300,000
		Switzerland	6,400,000
		West Germany	59,200,000
		Italy	54,500,000
		Spain	33,900,000

Portugal	9,700,000
Philippines	40,800,000
New Zealand	3,000,000
Australia	13,000,000
Turkey	37,600,000
Canada	22,200,000
and *all* of Africa	237,700,000

Total   800,000,000   *Total still not 800,000,000!*

Source: Latest available figures (mid–1971). Estimate from United Nations, cited Encyclopedia Americana, 1973 Annual.

As one reflects on the varieties of contributions made by the assembled populations of these many non-Chinese nations to art, music, government, science, medicine, food, fashion, architecture, war, literature—and notes that their combined population does not match that of China—then the potential influence of a China *in motion* has remarkable impact. If three million Irishmen have influenced the political habits of much of the world, what will two hundred and sixty-six times as many Chinese produce?

An analysis of the number of Chinese born each year compared to the total population of substantial existing nations is equally impressive. The estimated population growth in China is now 1.8 percent per year, or approximately 14.5 million each year. First of all, this means there are more Chinese born each year than the total population of the Netherlands. Even more arresting, politically, is the fact that this new population addition is almost equal to the total population of Taiwan, and more than that of Australia. And more than the population of Ireland, Norway, and Denmark combined. Each three years the new population in China is almost equal to the entire population of France, or Italy, or Mexico. The improbability of ignoring such a portion of mankind is apparent. When one adds to these numbers their energy, ability, and, now, *commitment*, the better part of judgment seems rapport—and perhaps a redefinition of our own commitment.

From the analysis, I reinforced what I already vaguely understood concerning the immense number of Chinese people. My thoughts did not turn to questions of the Yellow Peril or of a physical migration of these millions of people pouring out over the world. Instead, I began to think of the irrefutable force this mass of people would be if they began reaching out and involving themselves commercially, intellectually, and morally in the rest of the world. What an unpredictable but undeniable force China would be if *it* became missionary-bent!

Our plane landed at Athens, and we sniffed an hour of Greece and then went on to Bangkok. There we did not even leave the plane, but after thirty minutes flew on east, crossing Vietnam just below the demilitarized zone, and then turned sharply north. Fifteen hours out of Geneva, we reached Hong Kong. Such intercontinental flights never seem real. The combination of fatigue, blurring of the night and day, the mixture of passengers, all worth the best of Somerset Maugham. (Who are they? Secret couriers, devoted civil servants, Russians or Germans or Americans hurrying to build bridges and markets?) Too much food, drink you don't need, an airplane chair that reclines only to an unbearable angle. The remarkable 707 circling the earth every twenty-four hours. Flight 1 heading east in an endless circle of important unimportance. All of us in a hurry—but would it really matter if we all slowed down to ship time? Speed; departure and arrival schedules; tight time commitments building up tension. Would it not all happen as well at waltz time?

The strange suspended timelessness that absorbs one's mind and body has a useful effect, if captured, on one's thinking process. Thoughts quicken and move easily over time and circumstance. Ideas come fresh, and complications have solutions. If one can retain the sense of such movements, useful answers emerge. The problem is that of capture.

Late on the night of September 13, our phone rang in our room at the Mandarin Hotel in Hong Kong. Paul and Ina White, coming from the opposite direction, had made their long flight in from Boston. His voice was steady and full-timbred and I was relieved to know they had safely made the long trip and were in the same hotel in Hong Kong with us, and ready for our big adventure.

I first met Paul Dudley White when I was twenty-eight and he was sixty-one. It was at Massachusetts General Hospital, in Boston, and at that great old hospital Paul White had built the heart center of that time. His own career in cardiology is actually the history of cardiology. He had returned from the First World War after helping the Red Cross in Macedonia—his initiation in international friendship. Back at MGH, his chief persuaded him that the world of medicine was about to subdivide into special fields, and said that White would not be wasting his career if he concentrated on the heart. White had thought of becoming a pediatrician, but he finally gave in to his chief's advice and concentrated on the electrocardiograph, a mysterious new gadget already in use in Europe.

I arrived in Boston almost thirty years after White had accepted this challenge. In those thirty years, he had literally created a new field of clinical science. "Cardiologist" had become an understood label, and White's own textbook on the subject was the international reference book. In my time with him, I had become one of several score, all over the world, who took pride in saying they were "White-trained men."

When I left Boston, I took with me much that was more lasting than the 1948–49 details of how to treat hearts. I learned, or at least tried to absorb, Dr. White's remarkable enthusiasm and optimism. His system of managing his department left me marked for life. I have never known Dr. White to criticize anyone or listen to gossip or hear or see pettiness. His department and his environment appeared free of personal frictions. They certainly did exist, but no one could involve, provoke, or trap Dr. White into being a participant. He was removed from and immune from gossip techniques.

Modern psychologists press for ventilation sessions in which all involved can blow off steam and "vent their hostilities." There is a margin of merit in such advice, but at the same time there is a margin of merit in feeling constantly charitable about others. Dr. White mastered this impossible human control. He truly liked people, thought they were nice, that they were doing their best, that optimism was therapeutic.

Dr. White had another quality, which should be bottled, patented, and sold as a vital liquor. He had energy beyond compare. When I first met him, he was a traveling whirlwind, and those of us in training would laugh and say we'd been trained at his knee. His knee was what we saw as he went up the gangplank to catch a train or plane.

I was with him when he retired from Massachusetts General Hospital, and I was present at the farewell party. Many of us teared up at the remarks made that day in his office, and we felt we were seeing the end of a grand career. He was sixty-two, and all of us, in our naïve way, believed we were watching the old man fade away, and were overcome with sadness to think that this time had come to Paul Dudley White.

That evening, I was with one of the staff, Dr. Gordon Myers, and I told Gordon of my own gratitude at being in the last group ever to be trained by the old man and how affected I had been to be there at the end. Gordon gave me one of his famous large-eyeball expressions and said, "E. Grey, you have not discovered the real Paul White." I encouraged him to go on, and he phrased it this way: "Dr. White is an irresistible force. You are impressed with his kindness and his unwillingness to see or hear bad. You are missing the point. Dr. White sees and recognizes these things. He simply refuses to let them get in his way. He has goals and objectives that are more important. I have watched him for years, and I describe him to myself as an absolutely driven, energetic, dedicated, sometimes very self-centered person. The best analogy I can think of to describe his career is as a mountain stream. It began a long time ago and was a trickle of cold water at the top of the mountain. The trickle gathered in volume and in force as it came down the mountain. It became a pounding force that could not be stopped. When it met rocks, it went around them, over them, tumbled them aside, or ground them down. Nothing stopped the stream, and if something was in its way, it was either gathered up in the rush or passed by and forgotten. Today you and I saw the stream at a junction, but don't be misled. Dr. White is no "old man" ready to retire. There is a great velocity and energy yet to come. Dr. White has just passed by MGH. There are many great leaps and runs yet to come."

Gordon Myers' analogy was wonderful, and it has never failed me in the subsequent twenty-three years as I was tumbled and, at times, gathered up by this mountain stream.

When the invitation to visit China had come, I had been

determined to include Dr. White, but his primary concern at the time was how could he fit it into his schedule. When I called him with the news of the invitation, he told me that the September 15 date suggested by the Chinese made a long visit impossible. I asked him what his major conflict was, and his reply was that he had to be in Rome on September 27 to meet the Pope! We chuckled together over the eclectic kind of travel that would take him from Communism to Catholicism on the same tour.

The Chinese had indicated to me their concern in receiving the eighty-five-year-old visitor and their special apprehension over the state of his health and well-being while in China. Dr. White's recovery from a previous myocardial infarction seemed excellent, and he and I both felt that he would not be fazed by the China trip. But the Chinese still expressed concern, and I assured them that I would enter and leave the country with him and we would have adjoining rooms throughout the visit. I told them that, for better or for worse, I would assume responsibility for his well-being in China.

From the Chinese Embassy in Ottawa we had learned that two other American physicians were invited at the same time and that the Chinese planned to receive us as a delegation, although our objectives and origins were unalike.

Both of the other physicians were from New York City. Dr. Samuel Rosen, long associated with Mount Sinai Hospital, had received an earlier invitation from the Chinese in 1964. His skill in developing a superior form of surgical treatment for deafness had impressed the Chinese, and he had been invited to come and demonstrate this new surgery. In Rosen's autobiography, he describes the course of events and says, "The U.S. State Department put their foot in my mouth . . . and the invitation was withdrawn by the Chinese Medical Association."

I had never met Rosen or the other physician, Victor Sidel, whose special interest was in systems for health care. Sidel had studied the Russians' physician's assistant program, the Feldscher, and now was invited to China to observe the barefoot doctor concept. His contacts with Galston and Signer had facilitated his getting the Chinese invitation.

As soon as we arrived at the hotel in Hong Kong, I got in

touch with the China Travel Agency, the official organization of the People's Republic of China, and was relieved to find that they expected me, had all arrangements well in hand, and were prepared for us to cross the border on September 15. They also told me that Dr. and Mrs. Sam Rosen were in Hong Kong and were entering at the same time. The Agency gave me the Rosen's hotel number, and I immediately rang them up.

This was my first contact with Sam, and when I attempted to identify myself, it was obvious that he had not heard of me previously; more interestingly, he was unable to hide the concern in his voice when he learned that Paul White and I were also entering China. Sam and his lovely wife, Helen, had received their own invitation and, because of their bitter past experience with the U.S. State Department, had almost literally tiptoed into Hong Kong, hoping to enter China invisibly. But here on the phone was a total stranger who knew all about it, and, equally distressing, here was their first awareness that they were not going to have a great solo experience but that other American physicians were included.

This was my initial exposure to what I have since come to recognize as a form of China fever, or "I was first." This illness has many acute and chronic forms, and I have been guilty of my share. Usually it expresses itself in a straightforward sentence: "I was the first American reporter to enter China in twenty-two years." This key sentence changes only with the main descriptor: the first doctor, the first actress, the first senator, the first labor union representative, the first basketball player, and so on. At home in the United States, this becames a matter of elbowing aside one's friends and being "the first scientific organization to greet the Chinese in twenty-two years," or the first hospital . . . the first university . . . the first city west of the Mississippi and south of the Ohio . . . and so on.

In all fairness to Sam and Helen Rosen, their attack of "firstness" was very shortlived, and long before our visit to China was over we were able to understand and enjoy each other, to share the fatigue, the excitement, the turmoil, and to reach beyond ourselves in our common task of explaining China to the United States. Sam and Helen Rosen are very important people, because they are willing to fight battles for causes they believe are morally good.

Late on the afternoon before we were to enter China, the head of the China Travel Agency in Hong Kong came to our suite and had tea with the Whites and us. Mr. Lai is a relaxed, urbane man in his forties who has helped many a nervous visitor make the long leap from the Lo-Wu Station on the British side to Shum-chun on the Chinese side of the border. For an hour, he patiently tried to decompress us and make us understand we were not entering a dark, mysterious, dangerous land. Our own years of Bamboo Curtain obscuration had made China and "Mao's faceless millions" seem capable of opening up, letting us in, and quietly closing the door—forever.

Mr. Lai was skilled and effective, and on subsequent visits has been a thoughtful helper through the complexities of the border. As is always true in life, if you have been through an experience once, you are forever an "old-timer," and my four subsequent crossings have never caused the same fast pulse and tension. But the first time is a day to remember.

Chapter Four

NEON CHINA AND NEW CHINA

ᶜᵐᵐᵐᵐᵐ

ON THE MORNING OF September 15, 1971, we gathered our luggage and took the Star Ferry to Kowloon.

To enter China from Hong Kong was an all-day task. There was no great amount of work involved; all baggage disappeared at our hotel in Hong Kong and reappeared at the Tung Fang Hotel in Canton. However, the excitement, even apprehension, was exhausting, and when day was done and I saw that Paul White was still bright and vigorous, I began to feel confident that his strength was equal to the full schedule.

This day is also an experience in two Chinas. Until noon, one is in the British Crown Colony of Hong Kong and able to see cities, towns, villages, roads, and people, and at noon one enters the People's Republic of China and sees the identical people but very different cities, towns, villages, and roads. The border separates the same genetic material, the Cantonese Chinese, into two sociological experiments. Hong Kong is 99.5 percent Chinese, across the border 100 percent Chinese. The traveler sees the same men and women, under two governments, doing unbelievably hard physical labor with an energy and drive that Westerners have always found remarkable. The obvious prosperity of Hong Kong is in neon lights, automobiles, and merchandise. Slender Chinese women in the latest-style eye make-up, hairdos, minis, and pantsuits, and the men almost foppish in their Italian-French chic clothes. But not all Chinese women and men are in full fancy. Hung on the hillsides are shanties of the worst hell, and people in rags are not uncommon. On the streets there are beggars. Signs warn of the risk of pickpockets. Newspapers report the latest narcotic raid and the nightly sweep for prostitutes. Stalwart police are visible on every block, and areas of Hong Kong are off limits to visitors because of the crime risk.

Then you cross the border, and there you see a People's Republic of China soldier, in a green cotton uniform and canvas shoes, with an automatic rifle, and that is the last armed person seen throughout China. (But one. One night at 9:00 P.M. in Peking, we went walking and by mistake attempted to enter the national headquarters of the Chinese Communist Party. There was a single armed soldier there.) One sees traffic policemen, but no patrolmen, no evidence of any police activity.

As you cross the border, you stop seeing either affluence or extreme poverty. The litter of Hong Kong is replaced in Canton by miles of tidy roadsides and fields and millions of people who certainly are crowded and often poorly housed but have somehow eliminated drugs, venereal disease, and prostitutes. Also gone is the hand eager for a tip, gone is the possibility of theft or even losing anything.

The fact that it is the same race of people on both sides of the border, and that twenty-four years ago Canton was world famous for its pleasures and now is a tamed tiger, makes the experience ever more remarkable.

In Hong Kong, one hears rumors that a thousand Chinese or more per month slip across the border. One thousand out of a population of 800 million is not an impressive figure, but still any thinking person must ask himself what price has been paid to bring about the changes in China. What have been the sacrifices, and where is the hidden hand of power that brings about such discipline?

As we crossed the border, a serious woman about forty years old stepped forward and greeted us on behalf of the Chinese Medical Association. This was Mrs. Chen Huei-sie, whom we have since come to know well, as she accompanied us through the border on five trips. Mrs. Chen is a capable staff member of the Kwangtung branch of the Chinese Medical Association. She has made the railroad trip between Canton and the border perhaps five hundred times, always to escort medical delegations.

On this September 15, 1971, day she was very serious, and one felt her own tension in this assignment to greet the first Americans she had ever seen. Here we were, representatives of the invaders of Vietnam, the bombers of Hanoi, the anti-Mao, pro

Chiang Kai-shek capitalists and avowed enemies of her government. Surely we were dangerous. Present also was a representative of the Chinese Medical Association to escort us to Peking, and he too was tense and guarded.

We could communicate only through an interpreter. This young man carried a small handbag in which he had his Chinese-American dictionary, his little red book, and a notebook of phrases.* The three of them walked us from the border, on past the heroic twelve-foot-high white statue of Chairman Mao, past the last wall banner proclaiming, "Down with the U.S. imperialists and all their running dogs," past bookracks of Communist literature with the titles *Imperialism, The Highest State of Capitalism, Manifesto of the Communist Party, The Civil War in France, The State and Revolution, Long Live the Victory of the Dictatorship of the Proletariat!,* past huge photographs of Lenin, Marx, Engels, Stalin, and Mao. Loudspeakers blared the martial sound of "The East Is Red." This initial saturation of propaganda is impressive and agitating, at least in one's first experience. With one stride, one crosses an invisible line called the border and leaves a familiar world, even if exotic Hong Kong, and enters the communized world of Mao Tse-tung.

Our hosts seated us in a private reception room, and then I tried to break through the tensions and establish some form of friendly communication. The effort was made artificial by the need to transfer all thoughts through the willing but inexperienced interpreter.

The effort was also made stiff because we found ourselves facing the ubiquitous phrases of Mao Tse-tung Thought. Within minutes, I was informed that cooperative efforts were possible through "Struggle—Criticism—Tranformation." We heard of people described as "poor and lower-middle peasants." We heard

---

* During one of our visits, on the second day, the interpreter sat immediately next to me at a conference table. I was intrigued to see that he was working from a prepared typescript in English. The responsible member spoke to us in Chinese; the interpreter translated into English for us—from his prepared text. I drew no ominous conclusion that this meant we were hearing only the Party line, but instead suspect that our hardworking, insecure interpreter had simply preceded each of our stops with a visit ahead to find out what was to be said, so he could improve his performance.

of the need to "serve the people" and "stand on our own two feet," of "dialectical materialism," "the countryside," "soldiers, peasants, and workers," and that "traditional medicine is a rich treasure house."

The phrases poured out and, no matter what my question, I received another dose. Only now as I look back do I understand that these three people, with their dilemma of how to communicate safely with foreign devils, were taking the absolutely safe route of using only the officially approved words of Mao Tse-tung. Dogma was a secure response, similar to prayer in the presence of sin.

In my innocence I pressed them for an outline of our travel plans, and could learn only that we would be met in Canton by a delegation of physicians; we would rest overnight in Canton and fly to Peking.

That evening in my steaming hotel room, in my shorts in front of a red and white rotating fan proudly labled, "Diamond, Made in People's Republic of China," I reviewed the day's experiences and the major cultural shock we had experienced in Marxism-Leninism-Maoism. Edgar Snow was right. This immersion in the People's Republic of China was far better than any attempt by him to explain.

I reviewed the list of things I wanted to accomplish in the ten-day trip. My list was numbered:

   1. Medical Education
   2. Acupuncture
   3. Herbal Medicine
   4. System of Medical Care

I wondered how I could possibly learn anything. My spirits were low, as were Mary D.'s and the Whites'. The overpowering propaganda and our inability to communicate beyond Mao's slogans did not promise much for the rest of the trip. We seemed destined for a solid wall of Marx. Our every question had ended up with a non-answer. The oppressive heat added to our depressed spirits.

At 8:00 P.M., I dressed and went downstairs, out of the hotel, and into the dark, quiet streets. As I adjusted to the darkness, I realized that there was active bicycle traffic, people walking, and carts moving. I walked on for a mile and passed busy restaurants, families sitting outside their doors, people talking and laughing. I was alone, no one had come from the hotel with me. People stared and turned away, no one spoke to me, no one followed me. I returned to the hotel feeling better for the walk and a bit freed of the weight of propaganda.

The next morning, we were told that weather problems would prevent our Peking flight. None of us thought much about the change in plans and, instead, enjoyed the heavy schedule of medical activities that was immediately arranged. Instead of our tense companions from the border, we were constantly with physicians. The next day and the next day, we were told that the weather was bad, and again we stayed very busy in the Canton area. A party of Canton physicians became our hosts, and a reasonable level of professional communication became possible. The unexpected amount of time gave the Canton physicians a chance to demonstrate to us in depth their progress in acupuncture anesthesia. This chance to review patients, their records, their medication, the process of acupuncture anesthesia itself, all provided me with the beginning knowledge I needed. From this experience, I realized that Edgar Snow had been right, and that it was essential not only that an American physician come and see acupuncture anesthesia but that the message be somehow satisfactorily spread in the United States.

I began to build my information base and to get professional questions answered. There was no longer any doubt in my mind as to whether I was seeing hypnosis, fraud, propaganda, or fact. Acupuncture anesthesia was valid, and the job was to determine why, how, and when. The question was not one of politics but of how to remove the bias that could obstruct scientific analysis and exchanges.

However, there were questions of politics during those days of which we were serenely oblivious. We accepted the bad-weather explanation for our grounding in Canton. Only many months later did we learn that the planes were grounded *all over China* at the direction of the central government. A major palace revolt had occurred in the very heart of the Central Committee of the Chinese Communist Party, and the second in command,

Lin Piao, his wife, his child, the army chief of staff, the head of the air force, the chief political officer of the navy, all disappeared from the scene. A single Chinese plane crashed in Outer Mongolia and burned, and the occupants were assumed to have been the missing Lin Piao and others who had attempted to seize the government.

cans, who promptly and enthusiastically announced, "It's bad for your health." Practically every Chinese man in the room at the same time was lighting up, inhaling, and enjoying his cigarette. Cool, wrung-out washcloths were passed for all of us, perhaps a party of twenty-five, including physicians and wives, Chinese physicians, staff assistants, and interpreters, and all sat forward on the edges of their overstuffed chairs, each smiling cordially. One would have been void of sensitivity if he had not sensed the warmth of the spirit and welcome.

Then began a formal greeting in Chinese by Dr. Hsieh Hua, who, we eventually discovered, was Minister of Health. I use the word "eventually," because one of the difficulties in modern China is finding out who is in charge. The tremendous disruption in administrative ranks following the Cultural Revolution has left unclear, in many areas, who is in charge. In fact, even in later visits I found that the leading position, or top responsible position, was often vacant. This disruption has not only left unclear the method of administration in many areas, including medicine, but has also perhaps made some of the best talent unwilling to step forward and fill positions which have high visibility. I found repeatedly that the responsible senior person was often the vice-chairman, or vice-director, or vice-administrator, with the primary administrative position unoccupied.

A rapid review of the Chinese professional people in the room divided them into two categories. There was a very attractive group of senior Chinese physcans, men and women, who were wearing gray, blue, tan, or brown suits cut from good wool cloth in the familiar Chinese tunic style, and standing out clearly and separately were several men in rumpled green cotton army uniforms with red patches on the collar and green cotton billed caps pulled down squarely on their heads. Through repeated experiences, one gains an ability to recognize these individuals as the "responsible members." Whether in hospital, factory, school, or administrative office, these individuals are authentic, loyal, well-trained "cadres," or agents of the Chinese Communist Party. "Cadre" is a word with which I was not familiar until this time, but now I realize that it is this group of intensely loyal men and women who represent the personal instrument of administration of China, the strong administrative communication link operating to carry out the policies defined by the Central Committee.

Many of these men and women are in their late forties and middle fifties, and they take pride in saying that they were "at Yenan." They are the men and women, most of them of peasant origin, who joined the Communists, as young rebels, during the eleven years the Chinese government was established and operating in Yenan, Shensi province, after the Long March.* In the language of Communism, this is the leadership which has come from the proletariat. Since 1971, in subsequent visits, I have noted that most of these men and women are no longer in army dress but are also wearing the typical civilian street clothes. However, one has no difficulty in immediately recognizing the cadre. Of course, the task is usually made easy when one is received at any institution, because the leadership of all institutions, even though not always in army uniform, is still in the hands of these "responsible members." Their mission, following the Cultural Revolution, is to be certain that the reorganization of any given institution is being carried out along the lines directed by the central authorities.

One can recognize the cadre also because there is an air of confidence; he is physically strong and frequently just plain tough-looking. By tough-looking, I do not mean thuggish, but the air of toughness and the strength of sinew that come from his peasant origin, when he labored in the fields, and his years of combat with the Chinese Communist army. I also do not mean to suggest that the ubiquitous spread of these individuals throughout all of the administrative structure of China represents a gang of wardens who are keeping recalcitrant citizens in line. There is undoubtedly that factor, but also these are trained leaders who understand management psychology and technique and are efficient administrators. Their administrative responsibility is one of

* The accomplishments of the Chinese leaders *since* 1949 must be appreciated as an extension of the goals set in the first territory they controlled in 1928, the Kiangsi Soviet. Much of the top leadership, now very senior, had been together six years in Kiangsi, one year on the Long March, eleven years encircled at Yenan, three years in the final conquest of all China, and now almost twenty-five years as leaders of the People's Republic of China.

carrying out policy as it relates to Communist commitments, but in no manner are they effective only because of the threat implied. The cadre system is one in which considerable training is put into techniques of persuasion, encouragement, and moral behavior. Moral behavior, of course, varies in every society, but one is safe in saying the present Chinese standards are puritan indeed.

The cadre is often darker-skinned than the scientific and professional individuals. I do not know enough about China to know whether this is simply the result of long exposure to the sun, working in the fields, or whether it is possibly the result of centuries of a sequestered mandarin group dominating intellectual areas and a darker-skinned group in the peasantry. There are two other physical characteristics of the cadres. In making such remarks, I am generalizing far beyond my base of information, but nevertheless, from my own experience, I have been intrigued by these observations. I am referring first to the evidences of missing teeth and gold and silver bridgework. The party members, obviously, have in some part of their lives had experiences which stopped their dental care. Second of the physical characteristics is the deep staining of fingers from nicotine. Smoking is an accepted national enthusiasm in China and a trademark of long-standing Party members. Snow had told me that at one time Mao Tse-tung cultivated his own tobacco patch and that Mao was an intensive smoker. Evidently, this enthusiasm of Mao's had made smoking not only officially acceptable but almost a badge of membership.

To return to our airport reception room, after the friendly remarks of greeting by the responsible member, Paul White responded that we were there in friendship and to open up again relationships between the medical professions of our two countries. In these remarks, we all slid easily into saying "Mainland China" and "Communist China" and "Red China." It was only as I detected wincing that I recognized we were using painful phrases, and we quickly got on the right track and spoke of the People's Republic of China.

Dr. White pressed forward in indicating our desire for normal relationships, and said that there were fellowships waiting at Harvard College. This was greeted with a loud silence, and again we painfully realized we had blundered; we were guilty of old missionary tactics and were again thinking of the Chinese as a backward people and ourselves as the Western heroes coming to introduce them to the modern scientific world. We quickly recouped, Dr. White as rapidly as any of us, and never again during our visit did we make a similar mistake. It was immediately obvious to us that the People's Republic of China was standing on its own two legs and that any American coming with thoughts of picking up where we had left off in 1949 was unlikely to be effective. Within twenty minutes of our landing in Peking, we six Americans were well aware that we were talking to a peer group, not a backward group of scientists waiting for us to bring pearls from the United States.

This meeting at the Peking airport was the first of what became a very familiar pattern. All visitors to China, from famous to inconspicuous, whether first-time traveler or repeat visitor, find the "initial briefing" an obligatory performance that cannot be bypassed. These briefings have certain overtones of indoctrination and usually present a moment or two of Mao Tse-tung Thought. However, the briefings are also a necessary bit of protocol. Why this is true can be appreciated when considered against the whole of being a "visitor" in China.

First, there is no reasonable way that the majority of Americans can tour China in the same sense as they have long enjoyed Europe. In part, this handicap is due to the Chinese government's desire to control, supervise, and restrict the activities of visitors. An unrelated reason is that the Chinese simply do not have the network of travel facilities that make for easy travel in Europe or the United States.

Movement between cities is not easy. Paved highways are very few. Rental cars do not exist. No filling stations. No motels. Rail and air service are used heavily for domestic activity. Hotels are few and committed to the use of official foreign guests and the many, many meetings of Chinese cadres. Added to the lack of transport and lodging is the absolute muteness of most of us when it comes to spoken or written Chinese.

An interpreter is an essential companion. In time, the Chinese will produce a sufficient supply of English-speaking interpreters, but the long freeze in relations with the United States also resulted in a decreased emphasis on the English language. The restrictions on the enthusiastic traveler, formed in part by a lack of intercity transport, hotels, and interpreters, are magnified by the very restricted supply of vehicles for movements of tourists within the cities. Without a prearranged agenda, there is no possible way of producing enough cars at the right place at the right time. Without the interpreter, one cannot tell the driver where to go. When arriving at a destination (factory, school, commune, hospital), one cannot make his wishes understood without the interpreter. Thus, the inevitable combination of a well-defined agenda, a personal interpreter, a reserved car, an assured hotel room, a definite departure and arrival date, all become necessary essentials of getting about in China.

The well-defined agenda falls naturally in three parts: What do we do this morning? What do we do this afternoon? What do we do this evening? These three activities are interlaced with thoughtfully prescribed periods of "take a little rest." The day begins early, two to three hours are free at noon, the day is done by 8:30 to 9:00 P.M.

Is all this structuring done for the convenience of the traveler, or is it a diplomatic way of keeping track of the traveler in a gentle form of surveillance? My experience would make me believe that it is a mixture of both reasons, but principally an effort to aid both the traveler and the hosts to get maximum effectiveness from the use of time and facilities. I have had sufficient "unstructured" time, in which I have walked at random for miles and miles in Peking, in and out of stores and shops, on and off public transportation, in and out of barber shops, camera repair stores, medical supply stores, sporting goods stores, markets, bicycle shops, restaurants, private homes, public toilets, and so on, to feel confident that one is able to mix, come and go, without any semblance of police restriction, frantic interpreter, or public hostility. My remarks must be weighed against the time of which I write—namely, 1971, 1972, and 1973—and in the knowledge that none of my efforts in "roaming" was remotely likely to jeopardize China's "national security."

Movement by road over a matter of miles—between cities,

for example—requires authorization to pass through checkpoints. I gather that this requirement affects foreigners and Chinese alike and is one of the means by which the Chinese have practically eliminated crime.

Thus, from the moment of the original visa discussion on through the agreement on travel dates, port of entry and exit, cities to be toured, organizations and places to be visited, one enters into a continuous series of "briefings," which are in reality a civilized means of communication. This experience begins at the doorstep of an institution: smiles, handshakes, three-way compliments via the interpreter, unhurried walk to the briefing room, careful seating of guests and hosts by seniority, large overstuffed chairs, lace antimacassars, sometimes conference table seating. Always cigarettes, matches, tea from thermos bottles, usually wrung-out hand cloths, formal declarative welcome by responsible member, meticulous translation, recitation of the institutions's achievements, requests for questions. Well-mannered American compliments the responsible member, makes notes, tries to sort facts out of the mixed-in Mao credit lines, looks up, and is intimidated by large photographs of honored prophets: Engels, Marx, Lenin, Stalin, Mao. The more diligent American, who eventually will learn not to overpress, persists in asking questions beyond the comfort level of the responsible member.

The visitor is encouraged to state his wishes, to indicate what he wants to do. Often, the visitor is well prepared and has a formal statement of his specific, determined, "let's get beneath the surface" interests. After another round of three-way conversation, the visitor finds that he is endorsing the original plan of his hosts and wondering just what happened to his well-rehearsed agenda. In this remark, I am being slightly unfair to the Chinese. On all three trips, I have been able to do almost everything I requested. There have been three exceptions, and I can only present them as examples of what one may experience in China. On the first trip, I asked to go to the Great Wall and was told that a flood had washed out the road. Later, I learned that movement north from Peking on that specific day had been stopped because of the government's concern over the Russian border following Lin Piao's attempt to overthrow Mao. On my third trip, I

asked to go to Tibet, not really expecting an approval. A straightforward answer was given. Tibet is closed to foreign visitors.

My third unfulfilled request was to visit a traditional oriental
medical school in one of the provincial capitals. Here I ran into a
gentle series of postponements, varying from "on vacation" to
"new students and busy faculty," and in essence found myself on
the train to the next city, still never with a negative answer but
happily waiting for a return visit. The world has a remarkable
education coming from the Chinese in the full use of the arts of
diplomacy.

The United States is discovering modern China. With our
usual enthusiasm, we have produced newspaper coverage, magazine articles, television documentaries, and a flood of books, each
telling an observer's story of his view of China. One might criticize the sameness of each report and infer that all visitors to modern China are escorted through a closely defined route which has
been specially rehearsed and polished for foreign persuasion. Instead, I believe the reason for the sameness of the reports is that
modern China does have a cohesive, uniform administrative program carried out thoroughly through all of China, and that this
vast planned management, when added to the homogeneity of an
ancient civilization, results in the China viewed by all observers,
regardless of the visitor's itinerary. All visitors to modern China
report the same observations not because their view is officially
restricted but because no matter where or how you inspect the
People's Republic of China, it is authentically of one piece. There
is little doubt that there are certain cities, and certain factories,
schools, and communes, which are very much on the "tour" and
seen repeatedly by foreign visitors. However, I have maintained
an inventory of the institutions visited by American physician
groups. The scope and variety is impressive and surely a reasonable sample of what is being done in China today.

We six Americans in Peking in September, 1971, stayed at
the Peking Hotel, which was also a base for delegations from all
over the world as well as several American groups. The rest of
the medical world is evidently equally enthusiastic in its desire to
visit China. I have seen delegations from all over the world in
China, and in three trips have personally chatted with delegations

and groups from Algeria, Nigeria, Tanzania, Yugoslavia, Cuba, Argentina, Canada, Mexico, France, and Britain.

The dining room at the Peking Hotel is an especially good viewing point for seeing who is visiting China. Viewing is the essential contact, because the various groups stay almost completely apart, each clustered at its own table, and essentially there is no conversation between groups. The lack of conviviality is perhaps related to the two different political groupings which characterize visitors to China. One is a Communist or one is not, and those gathered in the Peking Hotel dining room are not about to run the risk of associating with an unrecognized Communist, or capitalist, or imperialist. At the Peking Hotel, these aloof, isolated circles of visitors give one an awareness of the several separate varieties of "friends of China." The Albanian delegation, dark-haired, serious, even dour, in shirt sleeves, looking the very model of the proletariat; the Rumanian delegation, in dark business suits, husky men and women, tending to be overweight; the Tanzanian delegation, shining black faces, well-tailored clothes with colorful scarves for extra flair; the Japanese delegation, all neatly dressed, neatly barbered, all looking like IBM middle management; and, everywhere, large delegations of Canadians.

The Canadian-Chinese friendship is evidently one with a high value rating. Canadians of every profession are touring China. This warmth owes part of its origin to the contribution of the Canadian surgeon, Norman Bethune, who joined Mao's army in the 1930s and who died in China. Bethune's selflessness and literal sacrifice of his life have been made a part of China's endorsed literature. Bethune is as well recognized in China as an authentic hero and foreign friend as was Lafayette in the early days of our own Revolution. It is safe to say that Bethune is a name instantly recognized at all levels in today's China. Most Americans would be surprised at the cordiality of relationship between China and vast other parts of the world. To bring it closer to home, the relationships between China and Mexico on our south and Canada on our north are excellent. We Americans are now having a new diplomatic experience involving our country and China, but we have not yet had time to absorb the finesse of China's efforts with Canada, France, Mexico, Peru, Chile, Tanzania, Zambia, Pakistan,

Mali, Nigeria, Libya, Egypt, Algeria, West Germany, Iran, England, New Zealand, Burundi, Sudan, Australia, Ceylon, Japan, North Vietnam, Cambodia, Burma, Rumania, Zaire, Cameroon, Yemen, Guinea, and so on. For many of us, these countries have no significance, and we have not even learned which name, in some cases, fits what bit of geography. However, the raw materials which they produce traded for manufactured goods from China is an increasing economic reality, which will become a critical factor in our balance of world trade. The information base of many of us in the United States has been arrested at the level at which we are aware that Communist China and Communist Albania are lonely friends in the Red world and that Russia abruptly pulled out of China and left the Chinese stranded, without modern machines, technology, and skilled technicians. This description of China's plight is usually combined with an analysis of how Mao has almost wrecked China's economy by his personal insistence on ideological assaults, such as the Great Leap Forward and the Cultural Revolution. We have equated technology and production as the important ingredients, and we have missed the successful installation of patriotism, pride, morality, and dedication. It is these latter qualities that are accelerating China's world influence beyond our present anticipation. The Chinese are citing their own experience as an example of "do it yourself" revolution and of moral reformation. Equally, they are creating a Chinese market using a "people's diplomacy" offensive.

Chapter Six

CONTROLLED FRIENDSHIP
AND FRIENDS

IN THE NEXT TWO WEEKS, Paul and Ina White, Sam and Helen Rosen, Mary Dimond and I were repeatedly aware of the small unit of history in which we were playing a minor role. Equally involved, after the fifth day, were Victor and Ruth Sidel. The Chinese Medical Association was our official host, and the secretary-general of the Association was with us at all points in our visit. The secretary-general, Hsu Shou-jen, now promoted to the Ministry of Health, is a shy, diffident man. He is not a physician but has been a staff officer of the Association for many years, weathering the Cultural Revolution. His counterpart can readily be identified in any large American bureaucratic organization. His task with us was not easy. The many professional medical organizations of China, the medical journals, the very medical organization itself had all been hard hit targets of the Cultural Revolution. All specialist subdivisions had been stopped. For example, the Urological Society, the Orthopedic Society, and the Cardiological Society, which are typical mechanisms for bringing together professionals of special skill to further their cross-communication, had all simply been closed down. All medical journals were similarly closed down. Medical meetings, whether local or national, had stopped. Medical, dental, pharmacy, and nursing schools all had been closed down. Our invitation was coincidental with the initial Chinese efforts to work out the most effective and, although not expressed to us as a factor, the safest methods of getting these critical communication and educational systems back into operation. I used the word "safest" advisedly. The social system of medicine is a conservative establishment. It had been hard hit by the deliberate attacks of the Cultural Revolution. The

Chinese Medical Association in September, 1971, was only beginning to feel its way back into business and was seeking answers to meet the demands of the government. The more prominent the medical figure, the more severe had been his personal experience. Sustained periods of Struggle—Criticism—Transformation had resulted, and many of the specialists had ended up practicing medicine for a considerable period in distant rural areas.

Our visit coincided very closely with the reappearance of many of these prominent physicians. The natural hesitation felt by them as they attempted to interpret their appropriate role in post–Cultural Revolution China was compounded by their need to interpret the correct level of hospitality to offer these first American physicians to enter China. They had been severely criticized for their behavior as citizens of the socialist state. Major charges had been that they were only interested in practicing medicine as specialists in the big city as a carry-over of the style they had learned from the colonial-missionary-imperialist-oriented medical schools (Yale-in-China, Pennsylvania-in-China, Peking Union Medical College). Now they were handed the dilemma of day-to-day fraternization with this delegation of American physicians. In September, 1971, the United States and China had not reached the accord which resulted in the Shanghai Statement of February, 1972, identifying the solution to Taiwan as a *Chinese* problem. In September, 1971, not only was the United States insisting that the real China was Taiwan, but, in addition, we were actively bombing very close to the Chinese southern border and continuing, as we had for twenty-two years, to campaign actively to keep Mao's China out of the United Nations.

These three issues—the Taiwan question, the war in Vietnam, and the admission of China to the UN as the sole representative of China—were major issues which were reiterated to us by senior government officials as barriers to further medical professional cooperation.

However, the secretary-general and the Chinese physicians assigned to the task of being our hosts made no attempt to politicize our visit. Our hosts were comfortable with medical talk and with careful, friendly, benign conversation, and at no point were we ever alone with a single Chinese physician. Without emphasis, it was apparent that comfort came with numbers and group conversation. These restrictions were not the interference that they might at first seem. For one thing, we were *all* insecure about our appropriate roles. Each of us was caught up in the mixture of anxiety and excitement associated with long-standing political confrontation between our two countries. What was our correct role as American citizens? What does a good guest do who is surrounded by Marxist dogma, who is aware of his host's insecurity, yet who is charged up to bursting with questions and curiosity?

Each of the eight of us handled this in his or her own way. Gentle, kind Ina White finally had to say to our hosts that she didn't think it was nice—in fact, not good manners—to put up signs castigating all Americans as imperialists and running dogs. Sam Rosen spoke out and said he was not confident that the Chinese claims of success in acupuncture in deafness had adequate audiogram documentation. Paul White spoke frequently of his hope that the Chinese would never give up their bicycles, but he did think they needed moderation in their use of cigarettes. I pressed, perhaps harder than I would have if I had had a little more experience, for more evidence of basic research in the Chinese work on herbs and acupuncture. I add the modifier that I would perhaps have done differently if I had had more experience, because I have since gained a more adequate understanding of how very shaken had been all science and scientific medicine from the pressures of confrontation in 1966 through 1970.

With repeated exposure, I think I now understand the overwhelming dimensions of the social changes in China. Slowed medical education and research were an almost irrelevant by-product in the over-all whirlwind. My mistake was to examine only that sliver that matched my career. Later, on page 57, I describe some of the details of the Cultural Revolution. In time, I recognized that I was privileged to have a first-row seat and was witnessing in medicine only a part of the largest social drama of our time, in which the cast is the entire mass of the Chinese people and the plot is the reshaping of their social structure. China became Communist in 1949, but the real confrontation between old China and new China was the Great Proletarian Cultural Revolution. In that context, herbs and acupuncture were hardly worth noticing.

Our personal hosts had been carefully chosen. The Chinese

physicians who greeted us at the airport escorted us through each day and saw us to our plane on our departure. Careful matching of host and guest had considered age, training in the United States, and special field of interest. Paul and Ina White, as the senior American couple, were escorted by Dr. Chu Hsien-i, dean of the School of Medicine, Tientsin. The next senior couple, Sam and Helen Rosen, were escorted by Hsu Ying-hsiang, head of Kung Nung Ping Ear, Nose, and Throat Hospital, Peking. The third senior, Mary Clark Dimond and I, were under the personal guidance and attention of Wu Ying-k'ai, director of the Fu Wai Hospital, Peking. This hospital is the national heart and lung center. Wu Ying-k'ai's mastery of the English language is total, and the years of separation of China from the United States had not harmed his vocabulary. Wu Ying-k'ai, now sixty-four, with a smile refers to himself as a foreign invader of China. His implication is based on the historical fact that the last Chinese dynasty was the Ching, or Manchu, Dynasty, which had invaded China from Manchuria and overthrown the Ming Dynasty. Dr. Wu is Manchu, and thus humorously refers to himself as a foreign invader.

One small thing about Dr. Wu that impressed me was his ability to point out immediately anyone of Manchu extraction. This ability he gradually transmitted to me, and it was with a degree of diagnostic glee that I became able to recognize the facial, head, neck, and shoulder structure of the Manchu and to distinguish them from the Han people. Such a reminder is perhaps a first step in making a Caucasian aware that it is only lack of experience that makes one subject to the chauvinism of "I can't tell them apart; they all look alike to me."

Wu had much of his training under Evarts Graham at Barnes Hospital in St. Louis, Missouri, in the years between 1943 and 1945. He became the chief resident in thoracic surgery there. Among his well-remembered friends are Dr. and Mrs. Brian Blades and Dr. Tom Burford. On each of our three visits to Peking, we have been personally escorted by Wu Ying-k'ai, and in April, 1973, he was a delightful member of our small party, traveling several thousand miles with us, and finally escorting us to the border between Canton and Hong Kong and sharing with us the infinite barrier of the invisible line over which I crossed and he, willingly, remained behind.

The fourth and youngest couple, who arrived just as our visit was over, Victor and Ruth Sidel, were assigned the companionship of the youngest Chinese physician, Dr. Hsu Chia-yü, Shanghai Second Medical College, Shanghai. Hsu is well on his way to becoming a permanent link between the physicians of the United States and China. Hsu was educated in Shanghai in the days of missionary influence and went on to his medical education at Pennsylvania-in-China, St. John's College in Shanghai. He became a physician just as the Communist conquest of China was completed and has lived his life in equal halves, the first in Chiang Kai-shek's China and the second in Mao's China. All of his life has been spent in that almost non-Chinese city, Shanghai, and thus he does not come from the peasant and rural roots which characterize much of the new China. He is an urban, urbane product of middle-class, capitalist China who began his professional career just as Communism became the standard for participation. Hsu has made the transition thoroughly and effectively. His competence in medicine, in English language, and in Mao Tsetung Thought makes him a logical and valuable Chinese communication link with the United States. I have been met by him on my three trips to China, as have Sam Rosen, Victor Sidel, Michael DeBakey, Jack Geiger, Tsung O. Cheng, and others, and he was also a member of the first delegation of Chinese physicians who came to the United States in November, 1972.

Our time in China on this first trip, in September, 1971, went by rapidly, and if we were not allowed to see the Great Wall, we at least saw the Ming tombs and the Forbidden City. At the end of the first week, at the Peking Duck Restaurant, the ranking physician of the Chinese government, Hsieh Hua, read a prepared statement which finally gave an official sanction to friendly relationship. This statement said:

Respected Dr. Paul White and Mrs. White,
Respected Dr. Samuel Rosen and Mrs. Rosen,
Respected Dr. Grey Dimond and Mrs. Dimond,
    We are much delighted this evening to give this dinner in honour

of our friends from the U.S. medical circles. First of all, allow me on behalf of the Chinese Medical Association and the medical circles of our Capital, to extend a warm welcome and sincere greetings to Dr. and Mrs. White, Dr. and Mrs. Rosen, and Dr. and Mrs. Dimond.

Dear American Friends! You have crossed vast oceans to come to visit China. This manifests your friendly feelings toward the Chinese people and your good desire for the restoration and development of the friendship between the Chinese and American Peoples. For this, we express to you our hearty thanks. We believe that your friendly visit will not only be conducive to the exchange of experience and comparing of notes between the medical circles of our two countries, but also will promote the mutual understanding and friendship between the Chinese and American Peoples!

Respected American Friends, we welcome you to visit China. In the past twenty years and more, New China has made some achievements in socialist revolution and socialist construction, and some progress has also been made in our medical and health work.

However, there are still shortcomings and problems in various fields of our work, including our medical and health work. It is our hope that you will kindly give us your counsel and valuable suggestions during your visit here.

Now I propose a toast:

To the friendship between the Chinese and American Peoples and the medical circles of the two Countries,

  to the health of Dr. and Mrs. White,
  to the health of Dr. and Mrs. Rosen,
  to the health of Dr. and Mrs. Dimond, and
  to the health of our friends and Comrades present here.

At the end of that dinner, I asked Hsieh Hua for a copy of his remarks and permission to publish them in the United States. All of our Chinese hosts heard him agree, and later Dr. Hsu Chia-yü said to me that "the remarks of Dr. Hsieh are very favorable indeed for prospects of good friendship." In a very controlled country, every nuance has a special meaning.

One of my Chinese friends expressed this "controlled" friendship in the following manner: "You know, Dr. Dimond, I consider you as my very dear friend and someone with whom I have great sympathy because your ideas and hopes are honorable, and in many ways similar to mine. My thoughts are often with you, and

I hope we may be together in the future. I would say you are my own very close personal friend, and it is the will of my government, that friendship will grow and we will work together. But you must also understand that if my government decides such contacts and exchanges shall not happen, then our friendship can only be in our minds and unspoken. I am first and above all loyal to my government, and all physical evidence of our friendship is a decision to be made by my government. In my heart you would, of course, have a warm place, but that is a personal friendship that must be secondary to official friendship."

My reaction to such a frank statement of limited friendship is one of both hedged sentiment and sympathy. As I interpret most of my American friends and their attitude toward international friendships, it would be fair to say that, under the flag of patriotism, most Americans generate or turn off friendships. Perhaps our form of national persuasion is more subtle. Most of us do not remember our controlled "friendship" with the Japanese people in the 1920s, our general assumption of their disloyalty, even when citizens, in the 1940s, and our enthusiasms of the 1960s and 1970s with sister cities and their gifts to our universities. We as a people are led by press and public leadership into our version of friendship inseparable from national policy. Without a doubt, there is a heavier hand of controlled policy in Communist China; there is no visible debate and no place for challenge. In that sense we are different, and it is that difference which my Chinese colleagues could not afford.

The present Chinese position is that such friendships are official, and the exchanges of delegations not only to the United States but throughout the world are energetically under way. This is expressed in China as using "people's diplomacy," and there is no doubt that the Chinese are masters in the application of officially controlled "friendship."

Hsieh's remarks were the official signal for which our hosts had been waiting. In the carefully regulated language of Chinese diplomatic communication, the words ". . . conducive to the exchange of experience and comparing of notes between the medical circles . . ." meant that the door was open. The next day, I queried the intent of the message in conversations with

Hsieh Hua. At that time, we agreed that "a visit to the United States by a Chinese delegation would be appropriate following a successful visit by President Nixon to China."

Our last night in Peking, the Chinese Medical Association gave a dinner for us at the Peking Hotel. This was a far more relaxed group than those who had first greeted each other two weeks earlier at the Peking airport. At that first greeting, there was a mutual good will that warmed us all but a mutual lack of ease in how to express it. More important, was friendship permissible or taboo? Through an unspoken understanding, we had found a tacit level of communication within which all were comfortable. I had also had enough answers to my questions on Chinese medicine and acupuncture to feel secure about the accuracy of interpretation.

The formal declaration of welcome by the Chinese Medical Association had been followed by a similar announcement in the Chinese newspapers. Now, on this last night, Paul White and I each were given a set of simple gifts which could not have been more accurately selected for our pleasure. We each received first an ancient Chinese medical textbook in which angina pectoris had been described and an herbal treatment recommended. Next, we each received a formidable plastic manikin, of modern manufacture, defining the sites of acupuncture and related meridians. Finally, we were presented with our personal kits of acupuncture needles. The manikin and needles were exactly the right combination for our Chinese colleagues to have chosen. Although their own style of medicine was as modern and so-called "Western" as our own, they recognized the logic and good sense of thus paying a degree of acknowledgment to "the rich treasure house of Chinese traditional medicine" as urged by Chairman Mao, in recognition of their government's official policy of "marrying" traditional and modern medicine. They were also sensitive enough to foresee our own pleasure in receiving such thoroughly oriental remembrances of our visit.

We left China together on September 27. The Rosens and Sidels remained behind for further travel.

Dr. White had been wonderfully healthy and vigorous through the visit. He had resisted the temptation to overeat and had frequently confined his morning or noon meal to a bowl of milk toast. At banquets, he would go through the ritual of toasting by appropriate words and gestures but carefully avoided alcohol. His avoidance of alcohol was not because of a dislike for alcohol but because, several years earlier, he had experienced an episode of herpes while visiting Schweitzer at Lanbaréné. Since that illness, which had affected nerves of his digestive system, alcohol had provoked intestinal irritation. Although this is Dr. White's analysis, I can only say that his drinking had always been moderate and, in fact, a bit innocent. I well recall my surprise when he responded to a host's query, several years ago, by saying, "Yes, I would love a drink. Could I have a full glass of creme de menthe?" Dr. White's sweet tooth included an enthusiasm for desserts and candy, which he soberly justified as necessary for the maintenance of his weight and strength.

In September, 1971, as we crossed the border into Hong Kong territory, Dr. White's strength, pep, vigor, energy, or whatever is the inner spirit, was in high gear. Not only had he got to China, but he and I knew we were seeing the door open and that the two countries were on their way to an understanding. He was in high good spirits and used the time on the train to the border to write a careful press release on behalf of both of us.

We knew we were facing a press interrogation. While still in Peking, we had received repeated telegphone calls asking if we were there as consultants to Mao Tse-tung. These calls had come from Los Angeles, New York, London, Dublin, Ireland, Kansas City, and Washington, D.C. Incidentally, the calls always came at approximately 3:00 in the morning. Neither of us could quite comprehend why such queries were coming to us, and we gave straighforward answers stating that we were unaware of any health problem involving Chairman Mao, but if there was one, the Chinese physicians were capable of handling it without our help.

We were still unprepared for the battalion of television cameramen and reporters with and without tape recorders who boarded the train at its first stop after the border.

One of the satisfying memories of that day which stay with

me was the sparkle and excitement animating Paul White as we became enveloped by press and photographers. His eighty-five years were indeed light upon his shoulders. The old man was 100 percent effective and handled the barrage of questions with wit, charm, enthusiasm, and gaiety. He was excited, but the lifetime of substantial public exposure gave him assuredness. I had followed him through the turmoil fifteen years earlier when he had faced daily press pressures during President Eisenhower's heart attack. Many Americans had then, for the first time, learned of a Dr. Paul Dudley White, and I can recall some who suggested he had been too outspoken in his willingness to define Eisenhower's daily habits. Those who knew Dr. White were annoyed then at the suggestion that he was an innocent among the sophisticates. The fact is that for thirty years before Eisenhower's illness, White was the dean of international cardiologists and had successfully faced powerful and sometimes irascible patients (and press) for a life-time. The enthusiastic and skillful response to the press on a Hong Kong train was simply the performance of an old war horse, charging forth once again to the welcome sound of trumpets and drums. Dr. White was a wonderful mixture of seasoning and youthful naïveté. His ability to handle the limelight and get "good press" sometimes left his colleagues grinding their teeth. This small number of detractors no longer existed, simply because Dr. White was the surviving member of the outstanding American cardiologists who first came on the scene after World War I. Survival to age eighty-five, and finally to eighty-seven years and five months, meant that his companions from the past had disappeared, but, equally, he found himself at the summit alone—and cherished.

At the Kowloon railway station, we parted from the Whites and they went directly to the airport for their flight to Rome. Dr. White had co-authored the translation of a Latin medical text which had originally been commissioned by an earlier pope. Now a presentation of the translation from the Latin was to be made to Pope Paul.

Chapter Seven

A REPORT ON
MEDICAL EDUCATION,
ACUPUNCTURE, AND HERBS

ON THE LONG flight home, I put my thoughts in order and reviewed the medical facts upon which I felt I could speak with reasonable accuarcy.

Thinking back to Edgar Snow and the primary reason for my China trip, I recognized the degree of jeopardy which was involved in any medical reporting to my American medical colleagues. This jeopardy had to do with the instinctive reaction of some of my more conservative colleagues, who would dispose of any report with the remark that anyone who had been to China was obviously a Communist or a Communist sympathizer. Remember, I am referring to the days when going to mainland China had not become a status symbol.

I recognized that any published comments I made would have to be as straightforward and as low-key as possible. Whatever medical reputation I had achieved over the previous thirty years would have to be my guarantee of reliability.

My visit had been brief but intensive, and there was no doubt in my mind on certain straightforward observations. The influence of Mao Tse-tung Thought, of a vigorous single national authority, the violence of the Cultural Revolution, the controlled press, stage, radio, art, television, the political theme of every presentation, was all there and incessant. However, there was also some impressive medical practice which American physicians needed to hear about. Even if they wanted to disregard it initially and, as one or two did, write letters to the editor suggesting that I had been "brainwashed," I felt that my reservoir of good will nationally among my colleagues would carry me through.

The impressions I had of the treatment of burns, of limb replacement, of deafness, of acupuncture anesthesia, and of potential new medicines from herbs, all convinced me that my task was to get the story told, to get a group of Chinese physicians to the United States, and to get more American physician observers to China.

On the plane, I began my campaign and composed letters to Hugh H. Hussey, M.D., editor of the *Journal of the American Medical Association*, the official journal of American physicians, and to Norman Cousins, publisher of the *Saturday Review*. Both replied promptly, and within ninety days my three reports were in the American literature.

The *Journal of the American Medical Association* used on its cover a color photograph of the Chinese acupuncture manikin presented to me by the Chinese Medical Association. This was a generous and important idea of Dr. Hussey's, and by late December I had a message from Peking indicating their pleasure. The Chinese sense of manners and correctness had not missed the significance of the appearance of their gift to me on the cover of the journal of the organizational counterpart to the Chinese Medical Association. After twenty-two years, the CMA and the AMA were in communication.

The twelve days in China had been full, and I had been able to have perhaps thirty hours of individual and group discussions with physicians and to visit the following health facilities: Kwangtung Provincial People's Hospital, Canton; Hsinhua People's Commune (hospital, dispensary, brigade, barefoot doctor), Kwangtung; Tungfanghung Kindergarten (infirmary, dispensary), Canton; Canton Deaf-Mute School, Canton; Fu Wai Hospital, Peking; Fan Di Hospital, Peking; Third Teaching Hospital, Peking Medical College, Peking; Peking Medical College (medicine and pharmacy), Peking; Textile Mill (hospital, dispensary, school, housing), Peking; Library, Chinese Medical Association, Peking; Library, Chinese Academy of Medical Sciences, Peking; Institute of Materia Medica, Chinese Academy of Sciences, Peking.

What the Chinese are doing and trying to do in medical education and medical care can only be understood in terms of the

population distribution of China and of the consequences of
the second, or Cultural, Revolution. The method of government
has been by a steady dedication to the teachings of Engels, Marx,
and Mao Tse-tung, a thorough application of communization.
From 1949 to 1966, this development of a single, a classless,
society moved, but in 1966, for a variety of reasons, a major
cleansing was launched. This sustained event, now officially desig-
nated as the Great Proletarian Cultural Revolution, continued as
a nationwide disruption for three years. The targets were essentially all individuals that we would identify as in management,
academic, professional, intellectual, or cultural roles. The students
were the primary arm of the government in this attack, functioning in a quasi-military manner, and university activity virtually
stopped. The government's encouragement to the students was
direct and can be quoted from the official Chinese book, *Official
Documents of the Great Proletarian Cultural Revolution in China*
(Peking: Foreign Language Press, 1970). The wording of the
following document also makes one realize how far removed life
in the United States is from Marxism. I cite those paragraphs that
relate especially to my own way of life, that of academic freedom, of science, of medicine.

10. Educational Reform

In the Great Proletarian Cultural Revolution a most important
task is to transform the old education system and the old principles
and methods of teaching.

In this Great Cultural Revolution, the phenomenon of our schools
being dominated by bourgeois intellectuals must be completely
changed.

In every kind of school we must apply thoroughly the policy
advanced by Comrade Mao Tse-tung of education serving the proletarian politics and proletarian politics and education being combined
with productive labor, so as to enable those receiving an education
to develop morally, intellectually, and physically and to become
laborers with socialistic consciousness and culture.

The period of schooling should be shortened. Courses should be
fewer and better. The teaching materials should be thoroughly transformed, in some cases beginning with simplifying complicated material. While their main task is to study, students should also learn

other things. That is to say, in addition to their studies, they should also learn industrial work, farming and military affairs, and take part in the struggles of the Cultural Revolution to criticize the bourgeoisie as these struggles occur.

11. The Question of Criticizing by Name in the Press

In the course of the mass movement in the Cultural Revolution, the criticism of bourgeois and feudal ideology should be well combined with the dissemination of the proletarian world outlook and of Marxism, Leninism, Mao Tse-tung Thought.

Criticism should be organized of typical bourgeois representatives who have wormed their way into the Party and typical bourgeois reactionary academic "authorities," and this should include criticism of various kinds of reactionary views in philosophy, history, political economy, and education, in words and theories of literature and art, in theories of natural science, and in other fields.

Criticism of anyone by name in the press should be decided after discussion by the Party committee at the same level, and in some cases submitted to the Party committee at a higher level for approval.

12. Policy towards Scientists, Technicians, and Ordinary Members of Working Staff

As regards scientists, technicians, and ordinary members of working staffs, as long as they are patriotic, work energetically, are not against the Party and socialism, and maintain no illicit relations with any foreign country, we should in the present movement continue to apply the policy of "unity, criticism, unity." Special care should be taken of those scientists, and scientific and technical personnel who have made contributions. Efforts should be made to help them gradually transform their world outlook and their style of work.

13. Communication of the Enlarged Twelfth Preliminary Session of the Eighth Central Committee of the Communist Party of China. Adopted on October 31, 1968

We must fulfill the great historic mission of the proletarian revolution in education. As regards intellectuals, they must be re-educated by the workers, peasants, and soldiers so they integrate themselves with the workers and peasants. The workers' propaganda team should stay permanently in the schools and colleges, take part in all the tasks of struggle—criticism—transformation there and will always lead these institutions. In the countryside, schools and colleges should be managed by the poor and lower-middle peasants, the most reliable ally of the working class.

The above directives have been carried out, and there is no way to discuss medical education and medical research in China today other than in a political context. The changes in medical education and medical care can best be described as a change in priorities. Between 1966 and 1969, the political leadership contested over this order of priorities, and the present programs are the result of the reaffirming of Chairman Mao Tse-tung's pogram and authority. These priorities are that medical care must be available *now* to all the people, not those in the urban areas only. The charge was made that too many physcians, university teachers, and scientists were not sympathetic to the unmet health needs of the majority of the Chinese people. Mao had used these words in criticism: ". . . it is the Ministry of the Health of City Dwellers. The expression 'Ministry of Health' becomes gibberish if it leaves 350 million peasants aside." An equal priority is that education (in this case, medical education) must be controlled by the people, not by an academic framework as we know it, and that entrance to higher education is earned by proof of one's thorough study of Communism, not by grades, academic achievement, or creditation.

A synopsis of the events from 1966 to the present gives some idea of how these priorities have been accomplished.

Essentially, all medical schools were closed. All students were graduated whether they had completed the full curriculum or not. At Peking Medical College, this number totaled 1,300. All of these graduates were given assignments where health workers were needed. In most instances, this meant in the countryside. Most of the faculty were sent to the countryside for variable periods of time, usually for nine months to a year.

Authors publishing in medical journals were criticized as examples of men bent upon self-aggrandizement rather than identifying themselves with the people (the masses, the proletariat). The more important the scientist, the more non–goal-oriented his work, the more often his name appeared in the medical literature, the more vigorously he was criticized. Intensive experiences in

Struggle—Criticism—Transformation were the lot of most of the medical and scientific leadership. Here is a direct quotation, to me, from one of those who had been through the experience:

"At first I could not understand. I thought I was doing the best work I could and was doing what I had been trained to do. In my special field, our hospital was doing very complicated work at what we considered international standards. Our group not only published regularly in good medical journals but we had been invited to several international medical meetings to present our work. In spite of all this, I was physically forced out of my office by the Red Guard and made to stand in front of my hospital while the charges against me were publicly announced. Giant posters were all about the building listing my faults, even criticizing the excessive quality of the material in my clothing. They criticized my travels to international meetings as pleasure trips. They criticized my concentration on one field of medicine and said that I had allowed my staff to become so specialized that we did not really serve the people, but instead collected data for our articles and for our reputations. These criticisms went on for days and I could not sleep, could not work, and was never without ridicule. My staff did not help me because they were either under the same criticism or they realized the risk if they were to take my side. The Red Guards demanded my removal and the government suggested that I be sent away to the countryside with a mobile general medical team and be given a chance to reconstruct my socialist understanding. I was sent to the lake area, almost one thousand miles from here, and was there nine months. We had to make our own bricks, build our own homes, grow our own food and prepare it. Our days were spent in moving from village to village doing general medicine and surgery and much of our work had to do with schistosomiasis. We did hard physical labor, we practiced medicine, we had long serious study of Marx, Lenin, and Chairman Mao. We organized classes and gave instruction to barefoot doctors, we helped improve the commune hospital, and I began doing a great deal of general work in my field. I had no reason to do any of my special work because, to my surprise, I found that which I was skilled to do was not a real problem in the daily life of the worker. It was this experience which finally made it possible for me to see what Chairman Mao had been trying to teach us. It was true. I had become a big city specialist and I was spending thousands of my country's money and using a large staff of able young people all for purposes that did not really serve the people. My nine months in the countryside did successfully 'wash by brain.' My body hardened, I became aware of the hard life of the peasant, I learned how he lived and how hard he worked and I learned what medical care he really needed and how little I was prepared to give him. It was a blow for me to realize that for most of his health problems, I could not do as well as the Chinese traditional doctor.

"At the end of nine months it was agreed that I had reoriented my thinking and I returned to my hospital. A People's Liberation Army doctor had come to be head of the hospital. I was his assistant but there were no problems. He is a very nice man. We were allowed to continue some of our special work, but we have now become a general hospital for all of the neighborhood around us. Our clinics are now staffed by both western and Chinese traditional physicians. We also provide neighborhood care in all of the health centers and our ambulances help move patients and take our staff to see patients in their homes. I would say that most of our diagnosis now uses western X-ray and laboratory tests but treatment is a combination of traditional and modern medicine. The traditional doctors freely encourage modern surgery and defer to it. Our medical therapy is a complete mixture of western and traditional medicine.

"I now see that the Chairman was right and that we doctors must first serve the people. Even research must take a second place until we are able to assure all of equal medical care. You see, we in China are a socialistic nation and we believe that all are entitled to equal access of food, shelter, clothing, and medical care. We have not yet reached that place and some of our poor peasants live unbelievably hard lives. The purpose of the Cultural Revolution was to get away from class distinctions and class privileges and to produce an equality. It is all very hard on me because I truly had never suffered and my family has always been prosperous. Through struggle-criticism-transformation I have

begun to understand what Chairman Mao was saying. It is hard
to learn, however, and I keep studying and try to improve."

My friend made these remarks as an answer to hesitant ques-
tioning by me. In China, one is greeted with friendliness and
wonderful manners, but one also knows there is a heavy government hand on all such transactions. I had no desire to create problems for my professional friend, and therefore my willingness to
persevere in getting facts was gentled.

My impression was that this had been a major disruptive
event in the life of medical teachers and practitioners, and that for
many it has become a reality for existence—but with no reasonable alternatives. However, this requirement of getting out of
their institutions, becoming actual first-line doctors and nurses,
getting personally involved in the way of life of the people,
getting physically reconditioned, had also become a stimulating
experience for many. From no one, in groups or alone, could I
detect the slightest criticism of this program. This steady support
of a major disruption of a social system is almost too good to be
true. Even the vigor of Mao Tse-tung Thought hardly seems
likely to have been this decisive. My intent is not to suggest that
this program has no critics, instead, I want to indicate that the
prevailing national policy *is* prevailing, and that at all visible levels
of action it is the accepted system. One can only assume or guess
that for many this has been a bending with authority and an
acceptance of something over which they had no control.

For a period of several years, there was no activity at the
medical schools, and then the administrative structure of the
medical schools (as well as *all* organizations: factories, communes,
primary schools, hospitals, and so on) was placed under "revolutionary committees." The revolutionary committee has three
kinds of membership. First, a representative of the People's Liberation Army. Second, a member of the masses, which means essentially a politically active and trusted worker or student. And
third, a representative of the administration or faculty. When one
visits a hospital or medical school today, the individual in charge
of this committee is identified as the "responsible member" and
is the chief administrative officer.

At the Peking Medical College, we were met by its revolutionary committee, and the army officer in charge gave us a detailed briefing of the present educational structure:

1) The medical schools have now been reopened, with first classes beginning December, 1970.
2) There is encouragement for wide experimentation with variations of the curriculum throughout the country, but within a framework of a total three-year course. Pharmacy is now a two-and-a-half-year course. These were six and five years previously.
3) Admission to the schools is from workers, soldiers, and peasants. Direct admission to college and on to medical school after high school is no longer accepted. Instead, medical student candidates are recommended or seconded by the revolutionary committee of the organization within which the individual works: factory, farming commune, or army. At the Peking Medical College, this new class, beginning December, 1970, numbered 360 students. The ages of this group vary from seventeen to twenty. Sixty percent are women. These students were selected by the following steps:
   (a) Individual wants to study medicine.
   (b) Recommendation by the commune, fellow workers, or military indicating that he has been a good worker, has identified with the masses, and is a bona fide proletarian.
   (c) Approval by the Party and confirmation that the applicant has thoroughly studied Mao Tse-tung Thought and is a bona fide proponent of Communism.
   (d) Individual is acceptable to the revolutionary committee of the medical school.

The responsible member of the revolutionary committee summarized the admission requirements with the brief statement that "they were all selected because they are good students of Chairman Mao's teachings." The responsible member also gave us the following information:

"Peking Medical College was founded in 1911. In its thirty-seven years before liberation the graduates numbered 1,069; in the twenty-two years since liberation there have been more than 10,000 graduates from the four faculties: medicine, pharmacy, public health, and stomatology. Before the Proletarian Revolution the curriculum was scholastic and repetitive. The method had been just like stuffing a Peking duck. Much of it was but dead reading. The physical health of the students had been poor because of the confinements of book education. This program had been cruel to the students. Chairman Mao said that the program must be shortened and must be of more 'essence.'

"The new three-year program combines Chinese traditional and modern medicine. This is true also in the school of pharmacy. The program uses the precepts of Chairman Mao: 'The student can teach the teacher, the teacher teaches the student, the student teaches the student.' Further, that education should be combined with productive work. Nurses who have had five or more years of practice may enter medical school and graduate as physicians in one year. There are 140 such students at the school now."

A general outline of this new curriculum follows:

Initial nine months: At the medical school, a coordinated course combining anatomy, physiology, biochemistry, Chinese traditional medicine, and political education. A second phase of this program coordinates pharmacology and microbiology in a lecture-laboratory course identified as Prevention of Essential Diseases. The microbiology class was visited, and this program consisted of studying throat cultures from two patients, working in the laboratory to identify the organisms, studying the effectiveness of various antibiotics on the organism, and maintaining a laboratory notebook. One could describe the course content as traditional but with a clinical orientation.

Two months: Military training, physical-fitness training, and manual labor.

One month: Vacation.

Six months: Lectures in clinical demonstrations and internal medicine, surgery, obstetrics, and gynecology.

Two months: Military training, physical fitness, manual labor.

One month: Vacation.

Nine months: Out to the countryside with their teachers

to do practical work. The medical school faculty and the students form mobile medical teams and in the daytime see the entire spectrum of medicine and surgery. In the evenings, clinical and basic science lectures are given by the faculty, using the classrooms of primary schools in the countryside. The students also receive formal instruction in the recognition, collection, and use of herbs and learn to use acupuncture. This is also the period during which the role of public health and preventive medicine is learned by on-job training. Students and faculty also engage in manual labor together, tilling a shared plot or doing road work, etc.

Three months: Return to the city for an intensive period at the university teaching hospital, which is to give students the chance to "consolidate what they have learned in the countryside." They are given lectures to complement their work and participate in ward rounds and clinical conferences.

Three months: A final three-month period in military training, physical fitness, manual labor, and vacation.

Upon graduation, each student will return to the unit which initially forwarded him as a student—to the army, the factory, the business, or the commune. Thus, the distribution of physicians will be general, based upon need and upon original source.

Repeatedly, we were reminded that the question of how best to prepare doctors, what to do about residencies, where the new faculty members would come from, how basic research would fit in, were all questions "undergoing discussion at all levels and that final decisions had not been made." A good example of this is the fact that none of China's own medical journals had been published for several years. This, too, is a question "under discussion," and just what role journals should play, which ones to print, how they were to be organized, and so on, were all being "widely discussed at all levels." Medical societies have also been tabled, and at present the Chinese Medical Association is the single organization. It, too, was attempting to define its right role, and no decisions had been made.

Schools of traditional Chinese medicine are active, and therefore there is evidently some lobby successfully promoting the uniqueness of traditional medicine. As a broad general fact, however, the new graduates of the medical schools will be considered as synthesizing the two methods of healing: Chinese traditional medicine and modern medicine. This same synthesis is now going on at all levels of care—from commune to the teaching hospital. Medicine and pharmacy as modern or Western disciplines are being used in patient care at the same time as Chinese traditional medicine. A patient with hypertension receives rauwolfia and acupuncture. A patient with angina has a twelve-lead electrocardiogram, a prescription for nitroglycerin and a Chinese herb ministration. A patient with chronic rheumatic valvular disease has a consultation with both a "modern" cardiologist and the consulting traditional physician; one orders prophylactic penicillin and the other an herb of reputation in preventing rheumatism.

With the major population mass in the countryside, the need has been to get medical care to the 700 million-plus people. The health personnel for this have been produced by a series of methods. As already described, one-third of the staff of all the medical schools and of all the hospitals must be in the countryside at any one time. This is not as discriminatory as it may seem; *all* urban dwellers, factory workers, students, army personnel, must also have a "countryside" rotation. This is a form of national "busing," with the objective of getting the city aware of the life, problems, and potential of the farmer. It is also undoubtedly a means of maintaining a revolutionary spirit, a sense of involvement, and grass roots orientation. Large numbers of well-disciplined high-school-age students, with knapsacks, can be seen hiking out of the city to begin their period of rural work.

The physicians are used essentially as professionals when in the countryside, but there is a requirement for a substantial amount of manual labor as well as participation in the political education classes. Professional duties consist of helping staff of the commune hospitals conduct continuing education programs for both health personnel and farmers, going out the individual farms and villages as model health teams offering medical and surgical care, carrying on active preventive medicine efforts, including sanitation, spraying, and vaccination, and training the first-line medical corpsmen known as the "barefoot doctors."

The barefoot doctors is best described as a combination farmer and neighborhood first-aid man. He or she has a minor dispensary at his disposal and acts as a first contact for the farmer and the connecting link to the regular physicians and nurses of the commune. Supervision of his work seems good, and efforts to strengthen his education go on continually.

One commune thirty-bed hospital visited by us serves 61,000 people and was staffed with regular trained surgeons, pediatricians, and general physicians. Consultants from the city also came on call. Urine analysis, complete blood counts, and blood chemistries were done. Modest X-ray equipment was available. This hospital made and sterilized its own intravenous glucose and saline preparations. A very large collection of herbs was maintained by the traditional physicians on the staff, and a pharmaceutical preparation shed was actively grinding, percolating, decocting, filtering, sterilizing, and labeling the finished product. This included the completed manufacture of sterile ampoules.

The actual collection of the traditional herbs is done in a variety of ways. I learned, for example, that a well-equipped pharmacy will have between eight and nine hundred crude drugs in stock, and a rough approximation of the source of supply indicated that 60 percent are bought, 20 percent grown in garden plots on the grounds, 10 percent actively sought for in the fields and mountains by the local staff, and 10 percent brought from overseas travelers.

All 61,000 people in the commune we visited have written health records. The barefoot doctor has the responsibility for keeping all vaccination and preventive medicine programs in motion. Birth control pills, birth control education programs, and abortions are all active elements in the program. The barefoot doctor's office was indeed simple. The essentials were there —battered, spare, but there. The telephone gave access to any needed level of backup help.

The need to maintain a large number of staff in the countryside has affected the work load of the urban hospitals. At one major chest hospital, the open-heart surgery schedule has been decreased from ten a week to two a week. A similar reordering of priorities was described at other hospitals.

In the city, the majority of births are in the hospital, often by a midwife. In the country, the majority of births continue to be at home.

The above description of a commune hospital is quite similar to the hospital of a large textile mill visited in the city. General medicine, surgery, pediatrics, obstetrics, basic laboratory and X-ray facilities, and pharmacy were available in this thirty-bed hospital. A large collection of native herbs and the production facilities for herb extraction and the preparation of sterile glucose and saline solutions were proudly shown to us, and the pharmacist gathered an aromatic collection for a photograph of Paul White sniffing among them.

In all health facilities, western, or regular, doctors worked together with traditional doctors. This is a fundamental requirement of the national health care program. In all health facilities—from the barefoot physician working in the peasant's home, to commune dispensary, to commune hospital, to municipal hospital, to specialty hospital, to teaching hospital—acupuncture was steadily in evidence, side by side with Western medicine. At the commune hospital, we saw a worker's hand with four previously amputated fingers successfully reattached, and in the next moment were shown a flask of brown liquid, made by the commune pharmacist, and advised that this brown draught, by mouth, was the best treatment for appendicitis.

The applied, or do-it-yourself, clinical pharmaceutical research now going on in China has an unpredictable potential. Much of it is not research as we know it, but is relatively unstructured day-in-and-day-out pragmatic clinical trial. One can only hope that the scientific skepticism of "Western" medicine acts as a filter, and that adequate data accumulate for documentation.

In this initial visit, I could not analyze the role of *traditional* acupuncture. By this, I am referring to the placement of needles at strategic points rigidly defined by ancient textbooks as specific therapy for either acute or chronic conditions. Major claims for this form of acupuncture therapy for the treatment of paralysis, bowel obstruction, migraine, deafness, and so on, were vouchsafed by my Chinese "Western"-trained colleagues, but again I have insufficient data. The instant interruption of an episode of rapid, racing heartbeat in himself was cited by one United States–trained Chinese "modern" physician. Still another "modern" physician emphatically described his personal experiences with migraine, in which ergot and Demerol were ineffective but acupuncture at three specific sites brought relief.

A safety control factor is that by government rule and professional discretion, all herbs and needling methods must be tried first, and adequately, on the prescriber himself. I have no yardstick for appraising the thoroughness of this self-control Food and Drug Administration, but the presence of such a requirement was cited repeatedly to me by both lay and professional contacts.

An entirely new application of acupuncture has been widely used in producing analgesia—so-called acupuncture anesthesia. This possible application is a real challenge to the physicians of the rest of the world. If true, the West needs to find new answers to some long-held basic concepts. If not true, then acupuncture anesthesia still deserves a reasoned analysis and explanation. Snow, Galston, and Signer had been impressed by this development.

On September 16, at the seven-hundred-bed Kwangtung Provincial People's Hospital in Canton, we were invited to watch and study three operations. Six patients were on the surgical schedule for the morning, three of the operations to be done under acupuncture anesthesia. We were given masks, caps, slippers, gowns, and full freedom of the surgical amphitheaters. Patients' charts and X-rays were at hand. The charts were of course in the Chinese language. However, the format was completely international: history, physical condition, medication orders, temperature, pulse, respiration, laboratory reports, X-ray reports, electrocardiograms, consultation opinions. Laboratory determinations were in Arabic numerals. Medication dosages and volumes were in the metric system. A reliable physician-interpreter was available. I will describe the first three cases in some detail.

The first patient was a forty-year-old-man with a large

tumor of the thyroid gland. On the night before surgery, he had received at bedtime 400 mgm Miltown. There were no preoperative medications. The patient walked into the operating room, took off his pajama top, retaining the pants, and stretched out on the operating table. One stainless-steel acupuncture needle was inserted in the front of each forearm, at a point approximately four inches above the wrist, at a depth of 1–1¼ inches, between the two bones. This point was carefully selected and identified as the most effective for anesthesia in thyroid surgery. A small bulldog clip was attached to the shaft of each needle and then connection made to a DC battery-power unit delivering 9 volts at 105 cycles per minute. Details of the wave form, current, and circuitry could not be supplied by the anesthetist. An intravenous drip of 5 percent glucose was begun, and to it was added 50 mgm of Demerol. Typing and cross-matching for blood had been done. During a twenty-minute "induction" period, surgical preparation and draping were done. No other anesthetic agent was added. The patient remained fully conscious and normally alert. He advised me, through the interpreter, that he was noting numbness and tingling of both hands; paralysis did not occur. After twenty minutes, surgery began, and a skillful team moved rapidly through the operating procedure. At one point, the patient took a sip of water. A large tumor approximately 2 cm by 3 cm was removed and the wound closed. The patient sat up, had a glass of milk, held up his little red book, and said in a firm voice, "Long live Chairman Mao, and welcome, American doctors." He then put on his pajama top, stepped to the floor, and walked out of the operating room. This considerable dose of propaganda was almost enough to convince us that we were involved in a large brainwashing hoax. All of us were fully masked, but I turned and looked at Sam Rosen, and he said a thousand words by simply rolling his eyes skyward.

The second patient was a slender fifty-year-old man with an ulcer of the stomach. The procedure was to be partial removal of the stomach. This patient had not had medication at bedtime the previous night. He was given 60 mgm Demerol in 500 cc of 5 percent glucose during surgery. Acupuncture anesthesia was introduced by placing four stainless-steel needles in each ear at carefully identified points. Again the needles were connected to a phasic DC battery source, this time 6 volts at 150 cycles per minute. Again the patient remained awake and alert, and chatted throughout the procedure. A partial stomach resection was done by skillful surgeons, scrubbed, gowned, and disciplined thoroughly in modern, or Western, surgical practice. This patient required no additional anesthesia but did note some sensation of tugging associated with manipulation of his intestine. No little red book finale occurred.

The third patient was a woman, thirty-five years old, suffering from an overactive thyroid. Her principal preoperative medication was an iodine solution, and she received an intravenous drip of this medication during surgery. Demerol 50 mgm was added to an intravenous drip. Acupuncture stainless-steel needles were placed in each forearm. These needles were not connected to an electrical source, but instead each was hand-manipulated throughout the operation. After twenty minutes of up-and-down plus twirling motion, the neck incision was made and a partial removal of the thyroid gland was effected without further medication. The patient remained relaxed and talked with a technical assistant throughout the procedure. The wound was closed, and the patient walked from the surgery.

Following these three operations, we had a detailed conversation with Chen Tseg-ming, M.D., chief of anesthesia. Dr. Chen is a modern, or Western-trained, anesthetist and has responsibility for the selection of appropriate anesthetic agent for all operations at this seven-hundred-bed hospital. During the lengthy question-and-answer period, he made the following points:

1 • They have now used acupuncture anesthesia as the anesthetic choice in 1,500 cases. The "success rate" in these 1,500 patients is 90 percent. By this, he indicates that sufficient anesthesia was obtained with only the addition of Demerol in a 50–60 mgm dosage. In the remaining 10 percent of cases, there was either a breakthrough in pain or insufficient muscle relaxation, and additional agents were needed.

2 • In 504 consecutive cases of thyroidectomy, acupuncture anesthesia had been used with 98 percent success, in terms of being the chief vehicle used for anesthesia.

3 • The first use in this hospital was in 1959, and originally only manual manipulation of the needle had been used. The introduction of phasic electrical stimulation was of recent origin. The electrical stimulation was solely to replace the manual burden on the acupuncturist. For example, certain surgical procedures required eight needles, and the manpower requirement for manual manipulation of this array of needles had complicated the use of the procedure. The introduction of the electrical stimulation had thus been a major labor-saving assist. The degree or rate of anesthesia was similar whether by hand manipulation or electrical stimulation.

4 • Dr. Chen did not want us to feel he was a proponent of "needlism." By that, he wanted to make clear that he fully recognized the role for spinal block, local block, and inhalation anesthesia. These he used when appropriate. He pointed out that of the six cases on today's schedule, only three used acupuncture anesthesia.

5 • Abdominal surgery was least satisfactory done under acupuncture anesthesia, because traction upon the intestines could definitely produce uneasiness, and also, strong abdominal muscles did not gain sufficient relaxation. In slender patients, as in today's case of stomach surgery, and with a gentle surgical technique, acupuncture anesthesia was adequate, however.

6 • Throughout surgery, the anesthetist carefully watched all usual parameters and maintained pulse and blood pressure records. Careful observation and conversation with the patient gave guidance as to the need for additional anesthetics. No attempt was made to "push" acupuncture anesthesia. Chen was simply convinced that it was a preferable form for obtaining patient comfort. He said that the merits of acupuncture anesthesia are that it is absolutely safe, that there is no interruption with the patient's hydration. The patient can remain on fluid and foods. There is no postoperative nausea or vomiting. The method is convenient and readily available. Chinese traditional physicians, skilled in acupuncture, added to the medical manpower available.

For example, in the case of the third patient, the "anesthetists" were Chinese traditional physicians. The procedure produced no lowering of blood pressure and was a very effective agent for debilitated or weakened patients. There were no postprocedure respiratory complications.

7 • Although the degree of anesthesia was greatest for the specific surgical site selected, there was also a generalized raising of the pain threshold. This was useful because if a cutdown was needed or a stab-wound drain placed, these could readily proceed with additional anesthesia.

To our question of how the acupuncture sites were chosen (both ears for stomach surgery), Chen replied that the sites were essentially those that had been traditionally established on the ancient acupuncture charts, but practitioners were now also identifying new locations.

Adequate anesthesia could be maintained indefinitely. He had had experience on difficult cases (brain tumor) of up to six hours. The duration of anesthesia persisted for several hours after withdrawal of the needles. If the patient had distressing incisional pain, a brief reinsertion and manipulation of needles would be used during convalescence.

The decision to use acupuncture anesthesia depended upon the full enthusiasm and acceptance by the patient. If the patient was very tense and frightened, a general anesthetic was administered, because it was not fair to the patient to have him alert and conscious during the surgical procedure.

Did Chen believe there was any element of hypnotism or autosuggestion involved? He laughed and said, "Obviously not." The method was being used in every hospital in China by literally thousands of physicians and upon hundreds of thousands of patients. Did we think everyone was hypnotized? If a severe fracture patient came to the emergency room, acupuncture anesthesia was routinely used, as it had been found that there was a much decreased incidence of shock. With such patients there had been no prior discussion; thus there was no question of autosuggestion.

Did he have any explanation for the mechanism of action? He

had no fully satisfactory answer but believed a neural pathway was involved. From his viewpoint, the total safety of the procedure and now more than twelve years of dependable results had made a scientific explanation not too important. Did we, incidentally, know how aspirin worked?

A week later, we visited the Third Teaching Hospital, Peking Medical College. This primary teaching hospital was built in 1958. It has 606 general medicine and surgery beds. There is a staff of six hundred. Since the Cultural Revolution, there has been a full coordination of modern "Western" medicine and traditional Chinese medicine. A prime example of this is acupuncture anesthesia.

The physician responsible for acupuncture anesthesia is a modern "Western"-trained physician, Chou Kuan-han. This institution has used acupuncture anesthesia since 1958, and to date has used it in 4,900 cases. It is used almost routinely as the anesthetic of choice in operations on the eye, nose, and throat, in chest surgery, caesarean section, skull surgery, limb surgery, and dental extraction. It is frequently used in abdominal surgery, but in heavily muscled men may not provide adequate muscle relaxation.

The surgical schedule for this day, using acupuncture anesthesia, was as follows:

Case 1: Woman, age forty; brain tumor; removal with adjacent part of brain planned. Condition of patient very poor.

Case 2: Man, age sixty-nine; removal senile cataract, left eye.

Case 3: Man, age thirty-two; unresolved pulmonary tuberculous lesion left upper lung; lobectomy planned.

Case 4: Woman, age thirty-one; left ovarian cyst; removal planned.

Case 5: Man, age fifty; chronic, recurent appendicitis; appendectomy planned.

Cases 6 and 7: Multiple tooth extractions.

We changed into surgical clothes and then observed the anesthesia induction and surgery on these seven patients. I will describe in detail three of the cases.

Case 1, the brain tumor patient, had received sodium luminal o.1 gm and atropine at bedtime the night before surgery. Mannitol 20 percent, 250 ml, was administered to decrease intracranial pressure. Three stainless-steel acupuncture needles were inserted subcutaneously. The first one was at the inner side, just above the left eye; the second was behind the left ear; the third was at the top of the skull inserted obliquely, right and anterior. Finally, a metal plate approximately 4 x 4 sq cm was attached to the back of the skull and a biphasic pulse generator attached to it and the needles. This instrument delivered 9 volts, from 120 to 180 cycles per minute. The patient was conscious but very weak. No other anesthesia was used. Respiration, pulse, and blood pressure were carefully monitored and recorded. All of the usual steps in opening the scalp and skull and removing a part of the brain were carried out uneventfully.

Case 3 was of special interest, as the patient was a modern, Western-style thoracic surgeon. Throughout his surgery, it was possible to visit with him and query him as to sensation and impression. A single injection of 10 mgm of morphine was placed deep, at a recognized critical acupuncture site: just posterior and inferior to the left jaw. One single acupuncture needle was placed in the left arm, at a point approximately midway between wrist and elbow, on the back of the arm. A Chinese woman traditional physician maintained steady up-and-down, to-and-fro rotation manipulation of the needle throughout the hour-long operation. A left chest incision, rib spreading, dissection, ligature, and removal of the left upper lobe were smoothly carried out. The patient-physician was comfortable but constantly querying his surgical colleague as to how the procedure was going, what were they finding, and so on. At the midpoint, everyone rested for a few moments while the patient ate some fruit. When the lobe was removed and free, it was shown to him and briefly discussed. We watched his face carefully as the incision was made and when the pleura was incised, but there was no wincing or facial change. His pupils remained equally contracted throughout the procedure. No other form of anesthesia was used except the single manipulated forearm needle and the 10 mgm of morphine. No special effort was made to assist breathing. I was told that in the days prior to surgery he had learned to breathe with one diaphragm.

(A year later, I saw the surgeon-patient by chance, sightseeing at the Great Wall. The recovery had been complete.)

In *Case 4*, Luminal 0.2 gm had been given prior to surgery. The acupuncture needle locations were complicated but essentially in two sets. First, two long needles were placed one on each side of the spine, approximately 3 cm lateral to the third lumbar vertebra. These needles were placed fairly deeply but obliquely, a full three inches of needle length. They were then connected to a 9 volt DC current. The curent was adjusted until regional muscle twitching could be seen. The patient complained of some discomfort, and the cycles were slowed from about 180 to 120 per minute. Next, three three needles were placed in each lower limb, one at about the midpoint of the lower leg, slightly medial; the second on the back of the foot at approximately the site of the midpoint of the instep, at the third toe; the third at the inner side of the juncture of the big toe to the foot. Identical placements were made in both lower limbs, and these were then connected to a 9-volt unit, separate from the one stimulating the needles in the back. Scopolamine 0.3 mgm was then injected at a certain acupuncture site in the right and left lower leg. This was described as a very efficacious site for this injection. (This was one of several times that I observed this rationale. In a case of slow heartbeat, isoproterenol was injected at a wrist point; in the cited chest surgery above, morphine was placed at a critical acupuncture point, and so on.)

Over a period of some minutes, the rate of discharge and amount of regional muscle contractions were regulated essentially by seeking the amount that was compatible with patient comfort. The final adjustment in the limbs was 9 volts, 0.25 amp, 120 cycles per minute.

After ten minutes, the abdominal incision was made and the ovary removed, the patient chatting throughout with the anesthetist. During visceral manipulation, the patient complained of pain, and Novocain was injected locally in the peritoneal cavity. An acupuncture needle was also placed in the ear at this time. The operation proceeded.

Following this, we had a long question-and-answer period

with Dr. Chou. We asked for more details concerning the electrical current characteristics. He apologized for not having more circuitry information, but explained that he was just an anesthetist, not an electronics specialist. He could say that their units were direct current, 9 volts, 0.5 ampere. The discharge rate could by varied from 120 to 180 cycles per minute; he assumed the contour of the wave form was a sine wave.

We asked how the anesthetist knew if he had placed the needles at the right point and depth. He said (and this same description was given at all seven institutions visited) that the patient feels a "numbness, distention, heaviness, and hotness" at the site, and if the wrist is needled, this sensation would extend into the hand, for example. Patients, he told us, occasionally were slightly sore at the needle site following surgery. Moderate bruising and black-and-blue spots sometimes were seen. He had used acupuncture not only for anesthesia but for pain relief in renal and biliary colic and in toothache.

He had not done research to determine basic mechanisms but appreciated that there are two schools of thought; one that there is a neural pathway, the other that the traditional channels as described by ancient Chinese acupuncture medicine are involved. He had made some observations. For example, following acupuncture anesthesia, there was an increase in white blood cells and a faster circulation time. There was no temperature rise. The material of the needles (steel, gold, silver) was not important. Novocain injection at the acupuncture site did not produce anesthesia at the distant point. Novocain infiltration widely around the acupuncture site did block the distant anesthetizing effect; he considered this evidence for a neural pathway. He had studied paired dogs, equally bled, and he was convinced that the dog receiving acupuncture at the appropriate site would recover while the untreated dog would die in shock. This research work was not yet in print. In cat, dog, and rat, they had found that appropriately placed acupuncture could produce sleep and a sleep-pattern electroencephalogram.

Dr. Chou said that he, as well as practically every "Western"-trained physician that he knew, had been thoroughly skeptical of acupuncture anesthesia and felt it essentially a hoax. It was only after repeated personal clinical experiences that he became convinced. Gradually, through guidance from his traditional medicine associates, he had learned how to carry out the procedure, where to insert the needles, and what were its limitations. He felt that it was simply a method that Western physicians must now recognize and that the basic research explaining the rationale would be coming along soon. For completeness and accuracy, I must record that in my description of the question-and-answer period I have filtered out a large selection of Marxist phrases including dialectical materialism and many acknowledgments to the teachings of Chairman Mao. Also, it completes the picture to add that an army officer, the responsible member, was present. My own interpretation was that Dr. Chou was a first-class physician, accurately describing his experiences with acupuncture anesthesia, and at the same time in the very tense position of needing to satisfy the critical eye and ear of the Party.

The next day, we met with the faculty of Peking Medical College and reviewed some of the classwork in the Schools of Pharmacy and of Medicine. We also met with two men involved in some research efforts to understand acupuncture. The work is being done along essentially three lines. The first is a study of the possible existence of some anatomical structure that would explain the traditional channels or meridians. A report from Korea had been checked by sending a team there, but it had been unable to confirm the Korean finding of a group of specially staining cells which seemed to be grouped at the well-known acupuncture sites.

Second, they were using electrophysiological techniques in rabbits, and by peripheral pain stimulation had produced a standard "induction voltage" in the cerebral cortex of 1–2 mm in height. Acupuncture when placed appropriately had proved to lower substantially this cerebral induction voltage, even though the painful stimuli application continued. They felt their preparation confirmed that acupuncture anesthesia did change the quantity of pain stimuli reaching the brain. Using humans and a standard stimulation of the tooth as the pain stimulus, they had found evidence that the recognized "tooth" acupuncture anesthesia point on the back of the hand, near the attachment of the thumb, would effectively eliminate pain stimulus to the patient.

The third research approach was of morphology and histology, especially of the ear. A cadaver study, in twenty instances, using injection techniques, had failed to demonstrate any special collection of blood vessels. However, special nerve staining had confirmed groupings of vagal nerve endings in the ear. One study now being done seemed to identify a very sharply localized collection of such endings, which when stimulated had changed the "electrical resistance" over the abdomen. They felt they were for the first time getting some suggestion of the possible neural mechanism for acupuncture anesthesia. These two men were Chow Chung-fo of the Acupuncture Department, Peking Medical College, and Dr. Li Chao-te, Department of Histology, Peking Medical College.

To learn about basic science research in other fields, we visited the Institute of Materia Medica in Peking. A component of the Chinese Academy of Sciences, the Institute has a department of pharmaceutical chemical synthesis, a department of phytochemistry, a department of pharmacological analysis, and a department of pharmacological research. The responsible member of the revolutionary committee is Kao Hsi-jung. The vice-chairman is Sung Ch'in-hui.

One active program at the Institute is seeking therapeutic agents for chronic bronchitis. Another section has done considerable work on extracting, purifying, and cooperating on clinical trials with an alkaloid Securinine from *Securinega suffruticos.* Very favorable results were described in the treatment of chronic paralysis following Bell's palsy. Results were also stated to be good in treating the paralysis following poliomyelitis. We did not see specific data, but were shown a number of before and after clinical photographs. The Institute team acknowledged that Russian workers had also tried this product, but in China they had not found the drug effective until they had increased the daily dose eightfold over that tried by the Russians. The course of therapy is one month, the alkaloid given by injection. They believe its effect is both in the spinal cord and at the junction of the nerve with the muscle.

A cancer chemotherapy unit was active in using tumor transplants in mice.

Another section of the Institute has successfully identified and followed into commercial production a rapid-acting digitalis glycoside, Neriifolin. This has been important because the crude plant grows widely in China and this has eliminated the need to import *Strophanthus-K*. The glycoside is extracted from the dried seeds of *Thevetia peruviana*.

Although ideological remarks permeated every conversation, the laboratories and the investigators were busy and productive. The work was thorough and substantial. I inquired about other institutes of the Academy and was assured they were all involved in basic research and "following the teachings of Chairman Mao." All are under revolutionary committees and all have the same countryside rotation program. These other institutes are: Industrial Hygiene, Cancer Research, Experimental Medicine, Epidemiological Research, Virology, Antibiotics Research, Hematology, Parasitology, Medical Biology, and Dermatology. (I visited the Institute of Materia Medica a year and a half later. A military officer was no longer in charge, and the tension among the staff had decreased. The constant citation of Mao Thought was lessened, and the staff was more at ease with an American visitor. Perhaps, too, the American visitor was a little more confident.)

Medical teams from the People's Liberation Army have provided staffing in deaf-mute schools. Enthusiastic claims of successful treatment of deafness by acupuncture need careful consideration. We reviewed medical records, including audiograms before and after acupuncture treatment, but my own ability to judge was inadequate, and the records we saw were incomplete. We did observe the acupuncture therapy as well as the superb speech therapy efforts. The acupuncture sites varied from forearm to below the ear to low back. The needle insertion was deep, brief (a matter of seconds), and, to my perception, painful. It would be wrong to discount or endorse this program without more information. The ideological indoctrination of staff and students at the school we visited was thorough, fiery, and impressive. Dr.

Samuel Rosen was also present and is joining the Chinese in a cooperative study, carrying out acupuncture himself in New York City and comparing similarly treated patients in Peking, using carefully calibrated hearing test devices. The Rosens work as a team, and both were in Peking in November and December, 1973, completing their study.

Chapter Eight

JOURNEY TO THE BEGINNING

ONE PERSON who was disappointed in my trip was Edgar Snow. We immediately called him upon leaving China. He protested that we should have stayed three months. We should have gone to Sian, Yenan, Hangchow, Shanghai. I could only explain to him my two time restraints, one being my commitment to the Chinese that I would personally guarantee Dr. White's well-being and escort him to the border, and the second, larger reason, that our new Medical School in Kansas City had just admitted its first class. I wanted to be in Kansas City and share the excitement. I assured Edgar that I would follow through and return to China. I discussed with him my medical impressions of China and my conviction that the Chinese had several technical skills of which the United States must be made aware. We also talked about the gentleness, the kindness, the thoughtfulness of medical institutions and professionals in China.

Within days, these last remarks became large in Edgar's life.

For several months, he had suffered from back strain and had tried various remedies. The problem would ease and then would return in a more persistent form. Finally, a clinician in Lausanne insisted on a thorough examination, and from this recommended exploratory surgery. I remained in close consultation and endorsed this approach. On December 26, in Lausanne, the surgery was done and inoperable cancer found. The immediate question was not further surgery, but the possible use of chemotherapy and intensive radiation. I called Dr. Ma Hai-teh in Peking, and in several conversations made clear to him the situation. Edgar's wife, Lois, kept in very close contact with both Dr. Ma and me as she began her role of maintaining Edgar's spirits.

Back in the United States, I wrote President Nixon and advised him of Edgar Snow's need for very special medical care.

My objective in writing Mr. Nixon was twofold. First, and above all, I was seeking access to the National Institutes of Health for Edgar Snow and the outside chance that something might be done to ease or help him. Second, and this I elaborated in telephone calls to the White House, here was a remarkable opportunity to show the world the errors of the tragic policy of previous years which had scarred the careers and spirits of honest men, such as Snow. Here was a chance to extend a humanitarian hand to an American citizen who had been right in his criticism of American policy. Here was a highly visible means of expressing to the Chinese leaders that the United States was indeed embarking upon a new policy in the Far East. Snow, a personal friend of Mao Tse-tung and Chou En-lai throughout their careers, if brought home for medical help by an act of the President, would be the human symbol of a changed policy.

The final White House response to me, by telephone, was to thank me for my concern and to advise me that the President could not make special exceptions . . . after all, there were many Americans living overseas.

Edgar received a letter, intercepted by Lois, which stated that the President was very sorry to hear of his illness and hoped for his recovery.

The response from China was somewhat different. Dr. Ma Hai-teh was instructed to assemble all necessary medical supplies, including hospital bed, intravenous fluids, medications, anesthetics, nurses, aides, attending staff, and senior cancer specialists. He was charged with taking the entire group to Edgar's home, and if Edgar was able to travel, to bring him and his family to Peking. If he was unable to be moved, the team was to remain with Edgar for the duration.

The group flew into Geneva and immediately took up residence at Edgar's home. Dr. Ma quickly recognized the final nature of Edgar's troubles. Consultative opinion between the Chinese and Swiss physicians and myself was uniform. We all agreed upon no chemotherapy, no X-ray, and no further surgery. The problem had reached the point where further attempts at treatment, other than comfort, would be meddling.

Dr. Ma summarized the effort, "We came to take care of

Edgar. We made his home his hospital and his hospital his home."

Chinese nurses assumed around-the-clock shifts of duty. A Chinese physician remained in attendance at all times. All food preparation, cooking, and chores were taken over by the Chinese. The Chinese Ambassador to Switzerland came frequently from Berne. Huang Hua, the Ambassador of the Permanent Mission to the United Nations from the People's Republic of China, came from New York City. Huang Hua had been Edgar's student at Yenching University and his interpreter when he broke through the lines in 1936 and lived with the unknown Communist leaders.

As the personal emissary of Mao Tse-tung and Chou En-lai, to convey and carry out their thoughtful concern for their old friend, came Ma Hai-teh. Ma Hai-teh (then George Hatem from Buffalo, New York) and Edgar first met at Sian in 1936 when Huang Hua and Edgar were waiting for their passage through Chiang Kai-shek's line into Communist China. The three slipped through together and remained friends throughout the following thirty-five years. The three old friends—one American, one American-Lebanese-Chinese, and the trusted Chinese Ambassador to the United Nations—gathered in Edgar's room. They referred to themselves as "The Three Red Bandits."

The end came on February 15, 1972. Edgar Snow, American journalist from Kansas City, Missouri, died in Nyon, Switzerland. His original analysis of Communist China, *Red Star over China*, is and will remain the definitive reference source for anyone seeking to understand the beginings and personalities of the originators of the People's Republic of China.

Mary Clark Dimond and I attended Edgar Snow's services in Geneva, Switzerland. No one present could avoid a shake of the head and a remark about the irony of timing and circumstances. The services for Snow were taking place at the time, to the moment, of President Nixon's flight to China. The journalist who had tried to tell his country its Asian policy was wrong, and who had brought personally from Mao Tse-tung the clear signal that Mr. Nixon would be welcome in Peking, left the scene just as American Asian policy made the giant turn away from the issues that had made enemies of the two nations.

A week later, as Mr. Nixon left China, the President and

Chou En-lai issued their "Shanghai Communiqué." This carefully written document defined the agreed-upon principles which would serve as the framework for future developments between the two nations. It was a significant document because, in essence, it spelled out the American government's acceptance of the end of its Asian Communist containment policy, the acceptance of peaceful coexistence, the withdrawal of our forces from Indo-China, the recognition that Taiwan is a Chinese problem.

No one in the austere John Knox Meeting Hall outside Geneva, listening to formal and sentimental eulogies by his friends, could help wishing that Edgar could have had his moment of satisfaction, following the bitter years. It is hard to see justice in such timing. Men want to savor their moment. The long years during which Snow painstakingly spelled out his observations and interpretations about China warrant more satisfaction than came to him at the end.

As the brief service ended in Geneva, Ma Hai-teh said, "Edgar was exactly what he claimed to be. A very thorough writer who worked hard at accurately reporting the events happening in China and trying for years to break through to the American people with a warning that American policies were inaccurately interpreting the course of events in Asia and Africa."

One suspects that tucked away in the luggage of every American—reporter, columnist, newscaster, President, wife, and secretary—in that exciting week in Peking was a copy of Snow's *Red Star over China*. They all, in the end, had to turn to it.

There is a more personal book by Snow which one hopes has been discovered by those who would like to review the origins of Chinese-American friction. That book, published in 1958, is *Journey to the Beginning*. This is a wonderful, warm human story of the young man from Missouri who made China his speciality. In the last pages of this remarkable book (remember it was written in 1958), Snow moved beyond journalism to the role of historian and said:

"No foreign policy ever attains all its aims. Even when aims are achieved, and seem to be 'right' at the time, the end result often turns out to be quite the opposite from that originally desired. Every power policy provokes an antithesis; the ensuing synthesis always reflects opposites and thus differs from both thesis and antithesis. We fought World War I 'to make the world safe for democracy'—in alliance with Tsarist absolutism. Probably the most important single change brought about in that period was the Russian Revolution. Winston Churchill boasted that he 'did not become His Majesty's First Minister in order to preside over the liquidation of the Empire.' Britain won the war—and liquidated most of the Empire. Stalin opposed the Marshall Plan and arbitrarily 'divided the world into two camps'; he frightened the divided west into a NATO alliance he wished to forestall. America imposed an embargo, an economic blockade against China, hoping to hasten the end of the Peking regime. To this challenge China responded by mobilizing its vast human resources as never before, in a rapid industrialization and educational program which strengthened China's economic independence.

"America cannot, of course, do everything in the world—alone. America's 'sins of omission and commission' may, indeed, more often be traced to a tendency to try to do too much abroad—and alone—rather than first doing the best possible at home. The awkward fact remains: 15 out of 16 persons on earth are not American and can never be expected to respond obediently to all the historical impulses which dictate our own policies. The rate of scientific discovery and overturn is so rapid now that within the next generation or so man is likely to advance, in an evolutionary sense, more than during the previous 7,000 years—if he can stay alive. In such a world, radical, social, and political change and adaptation cannot be prevented.

"Nationalism is not a particularly attractive phase of human development—especially somebody else's nationalism—but it is clearly an unavoidable transition towards regional organization, itself a step towards world order. The more every nation seeks to strengthen the United Nations organization, the more it focuses its means of communications with others—the more realistic a foreign policy it will have, and the less likely it is to be upset at coming reform and revolution still foreseeable in many lands on an unevenly developed earth.

"In this era, 'competitive co-existence' is not just a matter of persuading coy Cambodians or Arab oil kings or dictators to take dollars rather than rubles or Chinese money. It is equally a matter of developing attractive alternatives in our domestic life which will not only arouse admiration, but also which can be emulated by nations in a hurry—and all backward nations are now, or soon will be, in a hurry. No foreign policy is greater than the success of the domestic system which inspires it, and during America's pursuit of cold war aims abroad, grave questions have piled up in alarming proportions at home.

"Meanwhile, our journey to the beginning has brought us to the crest of an altogether unexampled flood tide of human advance, ready to carry forward nearly two billion underfed and undereducated people who are awakening to the new needs, new dimensions, new dreams of a future bright with hopes and freedom. For all of us today it is a time for every nation to cast out the beam in its own eyes before seeking to cast out the mote in a neighbor's eyes, a parting time from our pre-history, a true childhood's end when men at last have to begin behaving like Man."

That was Edgar Snow speaking at his best.

Edgar left behind another personal message, written before he became ill, asking that his ashes be cast, symbolic of his life and experiences.

"I love China. I should like part of me to stay there after death, as it always did during life. America fostered and nourished me. I should like part of me scattered over the Hudson River, to join other debris which touches our shores before it enters the Atlantic, and in turn touches Europe and all the shores of mankind of which I felt a part, as I knew good men in almost every land."

In late 1973, Lois Snow and their children began carrying out this bleak task of completion. A white marble marker on a campus knoll at Peking University reads:

IN MEMORY OF EDGAR SNOW
AN AMERICAN FRIEND OF THE CHINESE PEOPLE
1905–1972

Chapter Nine

PRIVATE CITIZENS AND
MEDICAL POLITICS

ON OUR RETURN home, I developed a formal paper on acupuncture anesthesia with supportive photographs and an hour-long audio tape and fifty color slides which have now been distributed by the American College of Cardiology to 1,000 physicians. I was determined to carry a message to as large a physician audience as possible. My message was to encourge the American physician to have an open mind about this unknown medical world, Chinese medicine. The new information about limb replacement and burn treatment was part of the message, but, equally, I encouraged an open mind about Chinese herbs and acupuncture. My concern was one of both too much and too little. On the one hand, there was the real hazard which would come from uncritical acceptance of acupuncture, moxa, and herbs. If the medical profession turned away completely and refused to give adequate study to these old and new ideas, then quacks, charlatans, healers, would quickly establish themselves as the purveyors of the procedures. The apt term "quackupuncture" was widely used to describe this cult. Through these months, I accepted all reasonable speaking invitations, and was before medical audiences in Chicago; Houston; Birmingham; San Diego; St. Louis; Indianapolis; Washington, D.C.; Ann Arbor; San Francisco; Scottsdale, Arizona; New York City; Omaha; Jackson, Mississippi; Waco, Texas; Columbia, Missouri; and Miami. In Kansas City, my wife was thoroughly involved with appearances before service clubs, junior-high and high-school groups and faculties, and produced a videotape and film-strip audio tape.

My aim was to provoke a response in the upper reaches of academic medicine and to generate a willingness to look at the entire question of Chinese medicine. I made clear repeatedly that I had no desire to endorse herbs or acupuncture uncritically, but urged research by the best institutions and visits by medical specialists in all fields to China as rapidly as possible.

I also made another decision which has proved useful, at least to my peace of mind. In spite of my curiosity, I decided to stay, personally, totally out of the acupuncture business. I use the word "business" intentionally. The American public has an immense, non-critical enthusiasm for any kind of therapy. Anyone with a quiver of needles and a white coat can undoubtedly make a fortune, quackupuncturing hundreds of enthusiastic patients daily. The truth is that most people would feel better for the experience. This is not necessarily because of any therapeutic success of acupuncture but because 85 percent of the ailments taking a patient to the doctor are psychosomatic. Such people enjoy attention and feel better whether the treatment is from a hollow needle through which a needless vitamin is injected or from a solid needle backed up by calm oriental inscrutability.

This decision to stay personally out of the field removed me from any commercial relationship and has been useful in helping me to maintain my objectivity and lack of emotional or fiscal involvement. I must admit that I smile ruefully over the thought that after thirty years of constant attention to my skills as a cardiologist, I could undoubtedly triple my income if I hung up my stethoscope and picked up my needles. Ruefulness grows when someone gently asks me if I am certain I would not help more people by doing so!

One of the early American reports about acupuncture came from James Reston's columns describing his gas pains and possible relief from acupuncture. His vast reading audience promptly flooded him with urgent requests for information about acupuncture therapy. With a mixture of both fatigue from the burden of the correspondence and a puckish sense of humor, Reston began referring all such queries to "the acupuncture authority, Dr. E. Grey Dimond." In fact, he used a photocopy reply form carrying this message. This Reston-launched flood of referral practice brought more than six hundred letters to my office asking for help. My only defense was to respond in a professional manner, defining my lack of skill and knowledge in the field and encouraging their continuing contact with their own physician.

Various requests from physicians and medical organizations requesting help on obtaining visas to China were stimulating but also frustrating. I was eager to help more American physicians inspect Chinese medicine, yet there was no official governmental link between the two countries. All contacts had to be through the Ottawa, Canada, Embassy of the People's Republic of China. In conversations with Peking, I was assured that "increased exchange of medical persons was encouraged." The Shanghai Statement of Chou En-lai and Richard Nixon had reinforced this intent and had removed barriers to further contact. The key word was "exchange." From conversations while in Geneva for Snow's services and by telephone between Peking and Kansas City, I recognized that the next move, in the minds of the Chinese, was ours. We had been there as their guests; now they were patiently awaiting an invitation to them, the "exchange" part of the understanding. I tested this idea with Peking and was assured that a suitable invitation would be favorably considered.

In the field of medicine, at that early period of changing relationship between our countries, because of chance and circumstance I was in a role which would not long continue. I found myself the acceptable go-between in medicine. Such a role was temporary and would rapidly end as others made contacts and friendships. However, from September, 1971, through November, 1972, I was involved in a privileged role as an acceptable negotiator and friend of China. The responsibility was significant and was complicated by the difficulties of distance and communication. The initial visit by the Chinese physicians was of critical significance. Their professional exposure had to be first class. Sensitive, thoughtful Americans needed to be involved. Contacts needed to be made which could lead to further exchanges. A friendly, happy visit was a critical end result.

Several American organizations were attempting to be brokers for arranging such exchanges. In fact, there was a degree of rivalry and self-promotion involved. All operated essentially from the basis of good faith, but there was also a considerable amount of individual and organizational aggrandizement. This same quality has shown itself in all of us who have been among the early venturers through the "open door" of new China.

I reviewed the American medical organizations and elected to approach two of them and ask them to join the Whites, the Rosens, the Sidels, and the Dimonds in inviting a group of Chinese physicians to the United States.

There is an organization, new on the American scene, which in many ways perpetrates a concept of elitism and clubiness I have always found to conflict with my concept of equalitarianism. Nevertheless, the Institute of Medicine, an administrative unit of the National Academy of Science, represents the best attempt of the United States to have a gathering place of academic medical leaders. The Institute of Medicine is in Washington, D.C., and, though authorized by Congress, it is not subordinate to governmental process. This last point was most critical in 1972, inasmuch as the Chinese were adamant in their unwillingness to deal directly with the United States government. In repeated correspondence and telephone calls to China, I tried to develop the point that the Institute of Medicine was quasi-governmental, not governmental. As to how that translates into Chinese, I do not know, but ultimately I had to go to Peking to clarify the point.

If the Institute of Medicine represents academic physicians, then the American Medical Association can be said to represent the private practicing physician in the United States. This seemed to me to be the logical pair of organizational partners to join us eight private citizens, the original doctors and wives who had been the guests of China.

The gathering of sponsoring organizations in extending an invitation was, of course, not the entire answer. Three major challenges to be met were: (a) what staff would handle the myriad details of hotel, travel, luggage, and so on; (b) what arrangements were necessary for security; (c) how much would it all cost and where would the money come from? Each of these problems fell into place. The first was solved, and solved well, by turning to a special committee of the National Academy of Science. This committee, the Committee on Scholarly Communication with the People's Republic of China, has an excellent administrative officer, Anne Keatley. Mrs. Keatley is the wife of Robert Keatley, of the *Wall Street Journal*, and the two of them had already visited China. Some of the early effective reporting in 1971 had been by Robert Keatley. In the spring of 1972, Mrs. Keatley's committee was a committee with a purpose in search of action. And action they were not getting. The committee's attempts to develop communication through the Chinese Embassy in Ottawa had met with silence. This was but a temporary stall; since then the committee has successfully hosted several Chinese scholarly groups, and finally has itself been to China.

Anne is deceptively petite, with straight brunette hair, a somewhat fatigued demeanor, a wispy voice, and a touch of iron that carries her beyond her seeming capacity. Earlier study in Hong Kong has given her ability in the Chinese language. Our common objective at the time was to further communication between the two countries. Anne, aided by Carol Rogers and Gwen Clopton, provided the needed staff.

The second need was some reasonable assurance of security and protection for the Chinese physicians. Our concerns were several, and they were shared by the Chinese. At best, the United States is not exactly a sanctuary of safety. Automobile accidents, murders, kidnapings, robberies, muggings, and bombings are all about us every day, and we have gradually adjusted our thinking until we almost consider such matters normal.

The Chinese simply do not have crime, at least as we would describe it. The reasons for this are several, but pertinent to my point is the fact that the Chinese do not have murders, hijackings, bombings, kidnapings, highway disasters, muggings, addicts, drunkenness, and so forth. This perhaps explains in part why their newspapers have so few pages.

Common thievery, such as the loss of a camera or luggage, does not happen to the visitor, but the visitor is not a reliable judge of what may or may not be the risk for the Chinese citizen. Most offenses which we now find common in the United States are evidently rare in China. As an alien traveler, I was impressed by my own personal safety and the safety of my property. There is a sense of good will toward one's fellow man when fellow man is trustworthy. This same feeling of security has been described by almost every China visitor. Small thievery, pickpocketing, and even break-ins may well occur, but the order of frequency seems extremely low.

In fairness, one must ask if the assault and destruction of people and property during the Cultural Revolution is not crime on the grand scale. My response would be that large-scale destruction in the name of public policy is called victory. A revolution, whether cultural or otherwise, is a crime—but only on the part of the loser.

To carry this further, the Chinese do not have airplane crashes (except the politically related attempted flight of Lin Piao to Russia, which is a very real example of the dangers inherent within the inner sanctum of government by conspiracy). Chinese planes do not fly if there is the slightest suggestion of rough weather. All travelers in China have had the experience of arriving at the airport and learning that they should go back to the hotel and come back tomorrow when the weather is good. Chinese commercial flights pay little attention to announced flight times. This is not because of casualness, but is related to the fact that the planes fly only when the sky is clear, the wind is calm, and all signs are good. Chinese flying is reassuring. Chinese planes do not get hijacked.

The Chinese themselves were concerned about the risk of daily "normal" violence during their visit to the United States, but they were also concerned over the activities of the Reverend McIntire, who had led rightist groups in picketing and placarding the Chinese table tennis team during its United States visit. Mr. Nixon's visit to China had exaggerated these differences, and right-wing groups were quite expressive in late 1971 and 1972. Demonstrations by Taiwan sympathizers had also plagued the table tennis visitors, and here, too, the Chinese wanted a degree of confidence before agreeing to send physicians. This kind of security was beyond the ability of any private citizen or organization, and I turned to the White House. The President's physician, Dr. Walter Tkach, was very helpful, and we obtained from

the President the commitment of a full detachment of plain-
clothes security personnel from the U.S. State Department. This
was a formidable and effective group.

Finally, where was the money to come from? Here the important help came from Dr. John Hogness, the first and quite
new president of the Institute of Medicine, one of the sponsoring
organizations. Although the security men were certainly govern-
ment-funded, we were anxious to pay all of the personal expenses
of our Chinese guests with private and foundation funds. Our
intent was to make it clear that the Chinese doctors were indeed here as guests of private citizens and non-government
organizations.

John Hogness is well over six feet tall, he carries a substantial
poundage well, and his face expresses kindness, friendliness, and
good humor. He quickly recognized that his new organization
could benefit by the visibility that would come with its assuming
the role of host to the Chinese physicians. He took over the task
of finding the needed money. We were not certain of the amount
of money needed, but realized that it would be considerable. The
group who had been the hosts for the table tennis team had raised
$100,000 and yet was still paying off debts. We assumed our
delegation would be smaller, and settled on inviting between ten
and twelve Chinese physicians and estimated an $80,000 budget.
Both figures proved too low.

Finally, in late spring, 1972, my wife and I invited Dr. John
Cowan, representing the American Medical Association, Dr. John
Hogness, and Mrs. Anne Keatley all to Dr. Walter Tkach's office in the White House and came to an understanding. (The
American Medical Association was hesitant at first about making
such a radical departure from its somewhat conservative policies,
but came around to seeing the logic in being one of the sponsoring partners.) I went directly from Washington to New York
City to the Chinese Mission at the United Nations. The proposal
was well received and endorsed but referred to Peking.

I returned to Kansas City, wrote out a letter to the Chinese
Medical Association, called my associates, Paul White, Samuel
Rosen, and Victor Sidel, obtained their approval, and forwarded
the letter to John Hogness with the suggestion that it go out

from the Institute of Medicine over his signature and that of Wesley W. Hall, the president of the American Medical Association.

On May 19, 1972, a formal letter was sent to the Chinese Medical Association on behalf of the four American physicians, their wives, and the presidents of the Institute of Medicine and the American Medical Association, Dr. John R. Hogness and Dr. Wesley W. Hall, inviting the Chinese to send, as our guests, a delegation of physicians to visit the United States.

Separate from these activities leading up to the invitation to the Chinese physicians, I had continued to press the White House through letters and telephone calls, and the Department of Health, Education, and Welfare through letters to Secretary of Health, Education, and Welfare Elliot Richardson, to Monte DuVal, Assistant Secretary for Health and Scientific Affairs, and to Robert Marston, director of the National Institutes of Health, urging that the American government move rapidly into studies concerning the basic sciences that might be behind acupuncture. It was satisfying to learn that finally a committee had been set up to study this area and that a million dollars had been set aside for the support of basic research. At the same time, the national epidemic of acupuncture was already well out of hand. In the complete absence of scientific explanation, an empirical endorsement of acupuncture had been made by the public. For better or for worse, the Bamboo Curtain had lifted—and the first items to pass through were ping-pong balls and acupuncture needles.

Chapter Ten

TO CHINA VIA ZURICH, SWITZERLAND

As soon as the letter was en route to China, a sense of calm and achievement should have steadied everyone involved. On the American side, the general commitment was made and little could be done in a final form until a response came from the Chinese. From the Chinese viewpoint, the Americans had made an appropriate response and the "exchange" invitation was in hand. Circumstances can usually find a new level of agitation, however, and this proved true here.

First, the invitation produced far more excitement in Peking than I had anticipated. True, a table tennis group had been to the United States, but now, for the first time since the founding of the People's Republic of China, a group of Chinese physicians and scientists would be guests in the United States. In extending our invitation, we had carefully identified all of those who had been our hosts in China, and our expectation was that it would be this group that would come. I had not reckoned with the nuances of new China. Our invitation did not bring a simple response, but, instead, all of the ingredients involved in the Cultural Revolution came into play.

Thus, the issues to be considered were not simply questions of who had been our hosts, or who was "most prominent," or who spoke English. Lengthy and sometimes excited discussions went on over a period of weeks with considerations of "reliability," "correct orientation of political thought," "correct attitude to the masses, the peasants, the workers, and the soldiers." These were the first yardsticks applied, but, equally, "the individual needed to carry the full respect of his colleagues." No insistence was made regarding Party membership, but satisfactory evidence of a serious attempt to apply Mao Tse-tung Thought to one's daily life was needed. Finally, a group of names was selected, and then other issues came forth. Was there an adequate mixture of all ages? Special concern was expressed that the group be essentially a younger group of active workers, with one or two senior members. Was there a reasonable show of female members? Was traditional medicine represented? Was there a wide representation of medical fields, and was the group representative of enough cities so there could be no criticism of Peking domination? Who would be the leader? Deputy leader? Staff? What would be the appropriate level of government involvement? Should an official of the Ministry of Health make an appearance? (I had included Hsieh Hua in the invitation, first because I like him and respect him, and secondly because he is the ranking physician in Chinese government.)

All of these very human and very political factors slowed down the official Chinese response to our invitation. Within two weeks of sending the formal invitation, I learned from Peking that it was favorably received, they would come, but it would take them some time to "make the arrangements."

Here in the United States, very human and very political factors were also at play. Our first crisis came when Dr. Walter Tkach and the White House overresponded to our request for help, and indicated with enthusiasm that the White House would be delighted to be the full host. This skillful finesse of what started out to be a private citizens' endeavor was, with good manners, turned down.

Our second domestic crisis developed around the role of the American Medical Association. Initially somewhat reluctant partners in hosting "Red China," they had come now to being very vocal in their demand for "equal time." Our original idea or hope had been to have the Chinese arrive in San Francisco at the time of the annual meeting of the American Medical Association, and that this would be their official contact with the American Medical Association. As time passed and no written response came from China, the AMA became more and more concerned, and finally insisted that the Chinese visit include a stop in Chicago and an official tour of AMA headquarters. This was arranged, and finally a formal schedule was produced that was still comfortably elastic, as we did not know when the Chinese were coming, when they would leave, who would come, how many would come, and where they would want to go.

Another minor concern developed at the Institute of Medicine, where the feeling was that they deserved a more prominent role and were not content with a "facilitative" role. After all, they had produced the money.

Another crisis developed in New York City. The two New York City physicians, Samuel Rosen and Victor Sidel, who had been paired in the Chinese mind as their "two American friends in New York," did not always see, think, or act in harmony. Although both lived in New York City, their daily lives were resolutely separated. In fact, their primary and only contact with each other had been in China, when pure chance had made them partners with Paul White and me. In New York, each operated from a hospital base, Rosen from Mount Sinai and Sidel from Montefiore. Competition developed between the two doctors and the two institutions concerning the Chinese. The enthusiastic wish to be involved in entertaining the Chinese physicians made planning both easy and risky. Every door was open, but, equally, any door we did not use was indeed sensitive.

Anne Keatley moved ahead with her staff work but essentially could not be definitive because of the lack of specifics. How could one reserve hotels and air travel in the absence of any information?

In July, Huang Hua wrote me from the United Nations to give a formal acknowledgment of the invitation and to suggest that the Chinese would come "after September 1." We, therefore all knew we could get on with other business until at least that date. I concentrated on my work in Kansas City through the summer, and in mid-August Mary Clark Dimond and I took advantage of a slack time at the Medical School and a house empty of children and took off for two weeks in Switzerland.

Our plan was to see Lois Snow and see if we could be helpful in any of the painful readjustments following Edgar's death. Shortly after his death, she and her sister had been escorted by George Hatem (Ma Hai-teh) to China. This was Chou En-lai's invitation and attempt to offer the always effective therapy of travel and activity. We found Lois in good spirits, working hard at sorting Ed's papers, in getting help to smooth out his unfinished manuscripts, in finishing her own book, *China on Stage,* and in hostessing the constant stream of old friends—and relative strangers—who wanted to know "how to get a visa to China."

The Snows' home is an ancient Swiss farmhouse, ceiling-high with books, the furniture a livable mixture, much of it Chinese and beautiful. To the right of the wall of books is a large color poster print of Mao Tse-tung, taken at Yenan in 1936 and displayed throughout China today. Unknown is the fact that the photographer was Snow and that the somewhat rakish cap on Mao's head was thrust there by Edgar a moment before the picture was taken. "Because he looked more military," Edgar would chuckle.

We took Lois to dinner in Nyon one night, and by an unplanned circumstance we were also the hosts of Owen Lattimore. He was on his way to China, and had come to see Lois to get advice and suggestions. My only previous contact with him was that of most Americans. I vaguely recognized that he had been one of those singled out by Senator Joseph McCarthy in the 1950s as a "Communist sympathizer." The power of innuendo and negative press had succeeded in casting an image in my mind of some devious and dangerous underground agent who had tried to infiltrate and weaken U.S. foreign policy. If such had been true in the 1950s, certainly remarkable changes have taken place. The Lattimore I met in Nyon (and later in Peking) is a mild, untidy professor at the University of Leeds, in England.

We left Lois and made a mountain tour of Switzerland. In the high valleys and along the wonderful walking trails, I was saddened to think of things and opportunities passed which cannot come again. To have a light pack, strong shoes, walking stave, lederhosen, time, and youth . . . and to be swinging along in the Engadine Valley . . .

I had made arrangements to be in Zurich, Switzerland, on August 28 and be ready to pick up on correspondence and phone calls from my office. After touching base, we were going on to the Black Forest, and planned to be home by September 7. Plans change quickly. Within an hour of our arrival at the hotel, the telephone operrator informed me of an incoming call from New York City.

Telephone conversations with Chinese Embassy staff are always impressive. They are impressive because of the very soft, quiet voice, because of the slow, relaxed pace of the conversation, and because the speaker usually does not identify himself. The conversation simply begins with straining to catch every word, wondering who is calling, and forcing yourself to slow down and give regard to the amenities. The call to Zurich was a classic, and immediately after it was over, I dictated a verbatim summary to myself.

EGD: Hello! Hello! This is Dr. Dimond in Zurich!

Unknown voice: Hello, Dr. Dimond. I hope you are well.

EDG: Yes, very well, thank you. And you?

Unknown voice: We are all well, thank you, although it is a little warm in New York City.

EGD: I am sure it is. I am sorry you cannot get away for a little holiday.

Unknown voice: There is so much to be done. The Ambassador has so many duties. There have been conferences in Panama and a trip to Peking. [*Pause.*] Dr. Dimond, would it be convenient for you to go to Peking? We have your visa here in New York City if you do not mind coming for it.

EGD: Go to Peking? I'm in Switzerland. When would you want me to go?

Unknown voice: Would it be convenient for you to go now? Peking has suggested September 1.

EGD (*slightly excited*): Today is August 28, late afternoon. You are suggesting that I return now to New York, get our visas, and immediately turn around, fly back to Europe, and on to China?

Unknown voice: Yes, would that be inconvenient?

EGD (*feeling exhausted*): Could you arrange for us to obtain our visas here in the Chinese Embassy in Berne, Switzerland? It would save time and money.

Unknown voice: One moment please. [*Long, long silence over the telephone wire, but rather animated Chinese voices can be heard in the background.*]

Unknown voice: Dr. Dimond? Sorry to keep you waiting. I have discussed it with my associates, and that will be quite good. Could you get your visas tomorrow? And then let me know your plane number and arrival time in Shanghai?

EGD: Yes, I understand. My wife and I are to get our visas in Berne, and we will try to arrive in Peking on September 1. I will advise you of my flight. Would you please advise Peking that I can only stay a few days?

Unknown voice: Oh? Can only stay a few days? How unfortunate. We were hoping you and Mrs. Dimond could stay for an extended time and travel widely. [*End of conversation.*]

Forty-eight hours later, as our plane refueled in Rangoon at daybreak, I stepped down on the tarmac and watched night watchmen and gendarmes awaken, scratch, urinate, wash, and yawn their way into another day of boredom. The steaming, wet fields and rusting sheds were hardly the Black Forest, where my planned schedule announced us to be at this time.

Chapter Eleven

SUBJECT: VISIT OF CHINESE
PHYSICIANS TO THE UNITED STATES

WE ARRIVED in Shanghai, stayed overnight, and went on immediately to Peking. There the usual sequence of amenities was pleasantly and solemnly followed. One has no way to estimate what the historical significance will be to our two countries as a result of their increased contact, but one can only hope that the Chinese sense of good manners and courtesy is one of the values received by the Americans.

The airport greeting was a convivial gathering of our friends. There in his Western suit, sports shirt buttoned at the neck, is Ma Hai-teh, and smiling gaily beside him is his Chinese wife, lovely Su Fei. There in the Western-cut suit, white shirt, tie, tie clasp, dark shoes, looking very European, dignified, happy, and serious all at one time, is Hans Müller. Beside him, in skirt and blouse, is his Japanese wife, Tsung Tsuen. Standing with hands clasped behind his back, with gray tunic suit, gray cap, tiny Mao button in his lapel, is Dr. Wu Ying-k'ai, head of the national heart and lung hospital. There is Hsu Shou-jen, secretary-general of the Chinese Medical Association. Bouncing up and down with gay spirits and a beautiful smile is the great obstetrician, Lin Ch'iao-chih. She is in pants and Chinese-style blouse, but there is definitely a touch of style and femininity. She hands Mary a bouquet and announces to all, "They don't approve of this kind of sentimentality any more, but I like it!"

The days went by quickly. Changes had occurred in the year since our first visit. Not large changes but modest suggestions of evolution from the stringencies of the Cultural Revolution. Last year, the head of every revolutionary committee at every school and hospital had been an army officer. This stage had passed. The revolutionary committees were still the top management unit, but were under civilian leadership.

The little red book of Mao's quotations had absolutely disappeared. A year earlier, it was in every hand. Peasants clutched it as we talked in the commune. It was beside each microscope as we toured the microbiology class at the medical school, marching columns of school children had waved it toward us in exchange of greetings. Part of the rapidity of disappearance of the little red book had to do with the fact that the preface had been written by Lin Piao and his photograph along with Mao's had been the frontispiece. The fall from power of Lin Piao had made the little red book obsolete, at least until the presses could be geared up to replace the estimated one billion copies already distributed in China. Try to visualize one billion copies of any book and the logistics of printing, binding, distributing, and getting rid of one billion obsolete copies at the same time.

Other evidence of a decreased emphasis of the need for public display of loyalty to Mao could be seen in the absence of Mao buttons on jackets and shirts. This button had been 100 percent present in September, 1971, and now, in September, 1972, it was perhaps 5 percent present. I asked about it and was told that the Chairman had thought it was being "overdone," and also that there was now a universal recognition of the great leader and such displays were no longer necessary. I asked Wu Ying K'ai why he still wore a tiny button showing Mao in profile, and his quiet response, ending further questions, was, "To show my respect."

Our six days were fully occupied. As another evidence of change, I was strongly encouraged to make ward rounds, meet with faculties and students, and lecture. In fact, in a five-day period, I gave seven major lectures on cardiology. I had come to China from a European holiday, and therefore I was without reference text, notes, or slides. As I constructed each lecture, I was reminded of how much we Americans have concentrated on technical equipment and special procedures in medicine. Repeatedly, I found myself aware of how we had become absolute world authorities on the ultimate refinements of medicine and yet how much more the Chinese had done in making medical care available to all of their people. The very nature of the social system in China has forced a leveling and distribution of medical services. Pecuniary measurements have been removed. Basic research has not been stopped but is far less in amount (and importance) than in the United States. The Chinese have made a reasoned decision that the item of first order is to get medical care distributed and thoroughly available. By the very nature of their strong central authoritative government, they have defined and enforced a system which begins with first-aid workers, available every few hundred yards over the entire country, backed up by communication and transport systems which move patients to the next needed level of care—from barefoot doctor to commune hospital to municipal hospital to provincial hospital and, when indicated, to national special care centers. There is no mystery in the system. The phrase "barefoot doctor" is a cozy, homey expression for the first stage first-aid worker. Backing up the barefoot doctor is the commune hospital. The commune hospital is Spartan, but babies are delivered, hernias repaired, teeth fixed—and all within easy distance of the family unit.

The big city hospitals seem bare to us because we have long grown used to bright colors and lighting, to carpets, drapes, color TV, electric beds, private bathrooms. If one can convince himself that these are not items that relate to better medicine or, in fact, even better care, then one begins seeing something else in Chinese hospitals. Among these differences is plenty of personnel. Plenty of nurses, technicians, doctors. Also there is an abundance of sharing. Patients helping other patients. Staff and patients talking over the hospital's strengths and weaknesses. And remarkable quiet. Chinese hospitals are quiet. In some manner, they almost seem empty. Empty not because of a lack of patients and staff, but because everything else is missing. Drapes, Venetian blinds, chair with ottoman, complicated space-age bed, television, vending machines, telephone, aides interminably clogging the halls as they drag out the passing of water pitchers and trays—all are missing.

My professional contacts during this week of early September, 1972, gave me an excellent chance to visit at length again with the faculty of the Peking Medical College. Here, too, things were different from the previous year. During my first visit, I had worked hard at learning what basic science research was going on in the field of acupuncture. I had been able to learn, but it had been an uphill battle and each bit of information had to be extracted. This year, all avenues were open. I was able to find full evidence that well-trained basic scientists, including neuropathologists, biophysiologists, histologists, and so on, were deeply involved in trying to find a rational basis to acupuncture.

There is undoubtedly a feeling, although not expressed, that the Chinese scientists want to find the scientific basis of Chinese traditional medicines *themselves*. Here is an area which is their own natural arena. For too long, all new scientific truths have gone from West to East. The Chinese would take pride in exporting some ideas of their own.

When West meets East in the area of medicine, interesting things happen. Staying also at the Peking Hotel was an NBC film team under Lucy Jarvis and facilitated by Audrey Topping. Lucy Jarvis and members of her crew were trying acupuncture for a variety of complaints. The director of the camera crew, Tom Priestley, had the calf of his leg needled for an ache in some distant region. I first learned of his problem by the familiar curbstone consultation route, Ms. Jarvis stopping by our dining table and commenting upon Priestley's inability to get around because of a heavy, swollen leg. I offered to visit him, did so, recognized the classic picture of acute thrombophlebitis from instep to groin. I had not heard at this point of his acupuncture experience, but as I persisted in seeking an explanation of possible trauma, he recalled a deep penetration of the calf of the leg a few days earlier by acupuncture.* In more professional circumstances, I would have made no comment, but instead I ventured the gentle suggestion that perhaps the acupuncture needle had set in motion the

---

* On my third visit to China, in April, 1973, a member of the American delegation was Bernard Lown, a very well-known American physician. Almost simultaneous with crossing the border, Dr. Lown's back began to ache, and by the time we reached Peking, he was leaning askew at a thirty-degree angle. With honorable enthusiasm, he accepted the recommendation of acupuncture. Thereafter, the entire American delegation snapped numberless pictures of the needled posterior of the prominent American physician receiving his daily treatment.

trauma which resulted in phlebitis. Neither this suggestion nor
that the diagnosis was phlebitis was popular with Tom, and I
suspect to this day he is using another explanation. Nevertheless,
after a couple of very uncomfortable days in his hotel room, he
willingly accepted care at the Capital Hospital, and with anti-
coagulants, rest, and elevation, rapidly recovered.

The day following our arrival, we were advised that Dr.
Hsieh Hua, the Minister of Health, wanted to come to our hotel
to visit. This was cast as a social call, but from the moment we
were greeted by him it was obvious we were to begin negotiations. He brought with him Dr. Wu Ying-k'ai from the Fu Wai
Hospital and Hsu Shou-jen, the secretary-general of the Chinese
Medical Association. Tea, peanuts, cigarettes, wet cloth, all occurred on schedule.

For the next hour, he quizzed me in depth. Was this Dr.
John Hogness a "friend of China" and was the Institute of Medicine an appropriate host? How do you pronounce Hogness? Was
the American Medical Association a reactionary organization?
Would they be friendly to Chinese guests? What arrangements
would be made for security? Would exhibitions of acupuncture
anesthesia be premature? Would the Whites, Rosens, Sidels, and
Dimonds be involved? What is a quasi-governmental organization? Hsieh Hua obviously was concerned, and it was these and
other questions which he wanted to discuss with me directly. He
repeatedly apologized for the long trip we had made, but felt
that friendship between our two countries was important, and in
order to make final decisions, he needed to know all this, and felt
more comfortable in talking it over personally.

This conversation was through an interpreter, and even with
a good interpreter one still wishes there was some better way to
relate to another human being. I like Hsieh Hua. He is about
fifty, strong, and very soft-voiced. I have seen him both in uniform and in street clothes; his exact title is elusive. At times he
appears as head of the Chinese Medical Association, at times as
the Minister of Health, at times as "one of the responsible members of the Ministry." He was in Mao's army during the Yenan
days and became a surgeon through training in the field. He
entered Peking at the time of the Communist capture of the city,

and he has been in administration ever since. Wherever I have traveled in China—Sian, Yenan, Cheng-chou, Wuhan, Shanghai, Chang-sha, Canton—the head of the regional medical administration is a Hsieh Hua man. At the end of the talk, Hsieh Hua asked if I would put in writing for him, in some detail, the specifics of our invitation. We agreed, and later Ma Hai-teh produced a reasonable typewriter. Long into the night, Mary Clark Dimond pecked, groaned, erased, pecked, pecked away, typing out my proposition and seven copies. The next day, we gave our letter to Hsieh Hua, met with him again, and discussed further details.

The following day, Hsieh Hua responded and accepted the complete invitation. From Peking, I sent a telegram to the Institute of Medicine in Washington:

PARTY WASHINGTON FIRST WEEK OCTOBER. INSTITUTE MEDICINE, KEATLEY, AMA ACCEPTABLE. DURATION THREE WEEKS. TEN TO FIFTEEN PARTY. STRESSING HEART AND CANCER. DIMOND RETURN USA SEPTEMBER TWELVE.

DIMOND

Within three days Mary and I were in Kansas City.

Chapter Twelve

BRIDGES OF MEDICAL FRIENDSHIP

༺༻

FROM CONVERSATIONS in Peking, I had realized that the make-up of the Chinese delegation was to be far different from what I had suggested. The contesting, the need for balance, the political realities produced a list of essentially all new names. Of the original names, only Lin Ch'iao-chih of Peking and Hsu Chia-yü of Shanghai were among the party.

But there was a party, a party of Chinese physicians, and they were just as excited as we were. In the party were:

Wu Wei-jan, head of the delegation: male, 52 years old; vice-chairman of the Association of Surgery, All-China Medical Association; deputy chief of surgery of the Capital Hospital, Chinese Academy of Medical Sciences.

Fu Yi-cheng, deputy head of the delegation: male, 54 years old; deputy secretary-general of the All-China Medical Association.

Lin Ch'iao-chih: female, 71 years old; professor of gynecology and obstetrics.

Wu Hsueh-yu: male, 57 years old; director of ENT and Eye Hospital of the No. 1 Shanghai Medical College; professor.

Li Yen-shan: male, 50 years old; attending physician of hospital under the Wuhan Medical College, Hupei Province; lecturer.

Chu Chuan-Yen: female, 41 years old; deputy chief of obstetrics and gynecology of Jeh Tan Hospital under the Chinese Academy of Medical Sciences.

Liu Shih-lien: male, 46 years old; assistant research fellow of the Chinese Academy of Medical Sciences.

Han Jui: male, 43 years old; assistant research fellow of the Chinese Academy of Medical Sciences.

Chou Kuan-han: male, 36 years old; associate director of surgery of No. 3 Hospital of the Peking Medical College.

Chang Shu-shun: male, 36 years old; doctor of the Peking Tuberculosis Research Institute.

Hsu Chia-yü: male, 46 years old; associate director of internal medicine of the Tung Fang Hung Hospital under the Shanghai No. 2 Medical College.

Chen Szu-chun: Third Secretary of the People's Republic of China, Permanent Mission to the United Nations.

Lu Tsung-min, secretary of the delegation: Foreign Office representative.

Wang Lien-sheng: male, 39 years old; physician and French interpreter.

They arrived in New York City by Air France on October 12, 1972. Dr. White came down from Boston, the Sidels, the Rosens, and the Dimonds were there. John Hogness and the AMA were there. Security was everyplace. In fact, for the next twenty-one days, my two principal pleasures were the company of the Chinese physicians and the security. Mary Clark Dimond and I stayed with the Chinese throughout the tour.

I had never thought through the advantages of real and complete security before. If so, I perhaps would have considered politics. To have "security" means you do nothing for yourself, nothing happens until you get there, everything stops, awaiting your pleasure. This includes items that are minor when viewed singly, but enormous when made a part of one's daily life. When one has "security," one does not wait for an elevator, it is there, occupied by a bright-eyed agent. It does not stop at other floors of the hotel. You do not lock your hotel room, because a security man sits at a desk in the hall twenty-four hours a day. Your automobile is not driven by you. It is driven by a security man, another security man sits beside him in radio contact with the motorcycle policeman in front of the car, and a security man awaits your arrival at your next destination. You proceed to the private dining room when the meal is ready, leave for the waiting elevator without paying the bill. Someone rather noisy comes nearby? For security, he is escorted away. Your luggage is under security control and leaves your room, sight unseen, to appear in the next city in the next hotel room. You arrive at the airport via special entrance, go to a lovely secure lounge, and board the plane only after everyone else is seated securely.

One special moment I remember was on the high-speed freeway which surrounds Washington, D.C. We were zooming along, and in the front seats two security men were speaking to their walkie-talkies, listening to the incoming signals through their ear gadgets. A police helicopter was overhead, all entrances to the Beltway had been stopped, a motorcycle policeman was ahead and another behind us. The leader of the delegation, Dr. Wu Wei-jan, smiled at me happily and said, "We don't travel like this in Peking." I tried throughout the trip to explain that our daily lives were somewhat simpler.

The visit of the Chinese physicians to the United States was a complete success. There were no unpleasant moments. No demonstrations, no dangers, no discourtesies. Our only problem was one of trying to do too much. How can you decide what to show and do in this huge, complicated country? Especially when the viewers represent the first to take a look in twenty-three years and at that moment are the initial eyes and ears for eight hundred million people.

Our schedule included Washington, D.C., New York City, Boston, Chicago, Kansas City, and San Francisco. This was covered in twenty-one days, and the only wry note for me personally was later, when reading a medical journal; a medical science reporter had written, "Dr Dimond somehow wangled a visit to Kansas City out of them."

To be thoroughly chauvinistic, Kansas City was a special high point of the trip. Even "security" could relax. In Kansas City, wonderful citizens came forward and took over the hostmanship. James and Marti Crockett, Ed and Abbye Cross, James and Vera Olson, Nathan and Lucile Stark, Homer and Alice Wadsworth, and William and Frankie Wu all got involved as a citizens' committee. The Chinese met with numbers of our medical students and gave their single professional lecture of the whole tour. In fact, one of the real problems throughout the tour was that we Americans had so much to tell, so much we wanted to tell, that we did not give the Chinese sufficient time to tell what *they* knew.

In Kansas City, we slowed the tempo, and Wu Wei-jan spoke formally on behalf of the Chinese Medical Association to the University of Missouri and, Dr. Chou Kuan-han presented a 16 mm color motion picture of thirty operations done under acupuncture anesthesia. This film had been prepared by the Peking Acupuncture Research team. Chou narrated, and Hsu Chia-yü translated into English. It was a remarkable film. A copy of it was made into a video cassette and turned over to the American College of Cardiology.

Acupuncture anesthesia is obviously one of the major medical projects which the United States must examine with an open mind. What degree of applicability is there to the American way of life? Is there a fundamental scientific basis, and can it be improved upon? How can one get a broadly representative team of American specialists to China in exchange for a substantial number of Chinese specialists to come here, and determine if the concept is exportable? Such is the next significant exchange which must happen. The large problem here in the United States is how to present a truly worthwhile demonstration of acupuncture anesthesia without its becoming a three-ring circus.

Not all things good on the Chinese physicians' trip occurred in Kansas City. High points that stay with one was a lovely dinner at Woodrow Wilson House in Washington, with James Reston toasting Wu Wei-jan, the Chinese surgeon who had removed the Reston appendix; the clown at the big circus in Chicago who came up among us in the audience proudly showing off his Mao button given to him by the Chinese table tennis team; Paul White, age eighty-six, at his home, encouraging the entire group to take a vigorous after-dinner walk with him; the Chinese Foreign Office representative accompanying the group, who arrived tense and concerned and was gradually thawed by the good will; the shopping spree on which the prime targets were thermal blankets and sewing needles; and, of course, the wonderful reunion between Hsu Chia-yü and his medical school classmate, Tsung O. Cheng. The two of them had graduated from St. John's

Medical School in Shanghai in 1950, and the one had remained and become a devoted, sincere physician and member of the Communist Party, the other had made the long step into Western culture and become a citizen and respected physician in the United States.

In their twenty-one days, the physicians were at the National Institutes of Health, the National Library of Medicine, the Smithsonian Institution, Capitol Hill, the White House, the National Acedemy of Medicine, Mount Sinai Hospital, Montefiore Hospital, Rockefeller Foundation, Harvard Medical School, Massachusetts General Hospital, Peter Bent Brigham Hospital, Abbott Laboratories, University of Chicago, American Medical Association headquarters, Cook Country Hospital, University of Missouri–Kansas City and its medical, pharmacy, and dental schools, Ford Motor Company, the caves beneath Kansas City, Wayne Miner Neighborhood Health Center, Model Cities Neighborhood Health Center, San Francisco Blood Bank, Stanford Medical School, University of California–San Francisco Medical School, Kaiser-Permanente Oakland out-patient clinic, Syntex, wine vineyards, the giant redwood forest . . . When did you last do as much in twenty-one days?

One unexpected pleasure for all was the arrival in Kansas City of Lois Snow, at the same time as the Chinese physicians' visit. Lois had taken on the arduous task of a large lecture tour, alone, throughout United States. We were able to bring the Chinese and Lois together with a bit of capitalistic champagne for a toast to all, in our living room. An exhibit of the writings and memorabilia of Edgar Snow at the University of Missouri–Kansas City library served as a setting for the formal welcome to Kansas City by Chancelor James C. Olson. Edgar's sister and brother-in-law were present to greet the delegation.

The trip ended in San Francisco, and, appreciating my own fatigue, I was appalled to learn that the Chinese were to continue as a delegation to Canada—and on to France. At the banquet that last night, I proposed a toast to all present, especially to the AMA, who were our hosts for the evening, and then I turned to the Chinese and said that I had somewhat the sentimental feeling of a parent who had had a great deal of responsibility during the growing years of a child and who suddenly realizes that he is no longer necessary but that the child is a man and beyond the parent's control. It was in somewhat that position that I now found myself. A small circumstance had given me an unusual relationship in the development between our two countries, and now, with the first exchange of physicians accomplished, the time was right and satisfying for me to propose this toast.

"To the friendship of the physicians of our two great countries—the People's Republic of China, the United States of America. May Medicine be a bridge to understanding—and peace."

Later that night, after the banquet, Wu Wei-jan, the chairman of the delegation, and I met in my hotel room and made plans for the next delegation to go to China. We agreed that the Institute of Medicine and the American Medical Association should go. Dr. Wu felt that that would be "good manners." He then asked if I would consider bringing a special team of teachers who would review recent progress in American cardiology. I agreed to set such a visit in motion. Over the next year, two more American delegations visited China, their visits directly and indirectly stemming from Edgar Snow's original contact with me. Such developments would have happened regardless of Snow or myself, for the time had come for the two countries to know each other. It was nice to be involved, however.

The first delegation was of cardiologists,* all members of the American College of Cardiology and sponsored by the Bureau of Education and Cultural Affairs of the U.S. State Department (a first), with the help of Dr. Richard Arndt.

Mary Clark Dimond was a special guest of the Chinese and brought with her a complete collection of the writings of Edgar

---

* *Eliot Corday, M.D.,* Cedars-Sinai Hospital, Los Angeles, California; *E. Grey Dimond, M.D.,* University of Missouri–Kansas City School of Medicine, Kansas City, Missouri; *Donald Effler, M.D.,* Cleveland Clinic, Cleveland, Ohio; *Arnold Katz, M.D.,* Mt. Sinai School of Medicine, New York City; *Suzanne Knoebel, M.D.,* University of Indiana Medical Center, Indianapolis, Indiana; *Bernard Lown, M.D.,* Peter Bent Brigham Hospital, Boston, Massachusetts; *Abraham Rudolph, M.D.,* University of California–San Francisco, San Francisco, California; *Jeremy Swan, M.D.,* Cedars-Sinai Hospital, Los Angeles, California; *William Steinhardt,* staff officer, University of Missouri–Kansas City, Kansas City, Missouri.

Snow as a gift to the Chinese government. This visit was from April 22 to May 9, and Mary and I remained for an additional two weeks.

In June, the delegation * from the Institute of Medicine was received, and thus the first reciprocal visit was accomplished. This group was in China from June 15 to July 6, 1973.

In October, just one year after the Chinese visit to the United States, the American Medical Association was invited to China; this slow, deliberate cadence of a response every six to twelve months seems to be the rate at which the Chinese government is willing to move toward further exchanges. The AMA delegation was invited to China from October 20 to November 10, 1973.

The AMA responded with enthusiasm to the invitation, and all plans were going well until a cablegram arrived at the AMA headquarters on September 5, 1973, politely indicating that owing to "complications" in Peking the visit should be postponed until 1974 and the Chinese Medical Association would approach the AMA when the visit would be more convenient. This postponement, just six weeks before the expected departure date, was indeed distressing to the AMA, but is a prime example of the unpredictable range of negotiations with the Chinese government and the feeling experienced by all would-be travelers of speaking to a sphinx and receiving answers from a nameless void. The unpredictability of a visit to China, as demonstrated by the AMA experience, is one of the very good reasons why a traveler is well advised to announce his visit *after* he is in China.

Many other American physicians were in China in these first two years, famous, not famous, right, left, and center in

* Dr. and Mrs. John R. Hogness, president, Institute of Medicine; Dr. and Mrs. Walsh McDermott, Cornell University Medical College, New York; John J. Bonica, M.D., University Hospital, Seattle, Washington; Martin Cherkasky, M.D., Montefiore Hospital, Bronx, New York; John I. Ingle, D.D.S., Institute of Medicine; Seymour S. Kety, M.D., Massachusetts General Hospital, Boston; Philip R. Lee, M.D., University of California–San Francisco; Mrs. Ruth Watson Lubic, M.A., C.N.M., Maternity Center Association, New York; George I. Lythcott, M.D., College of Physicians and Surgeons, Columbia University, New York; Leo A. Orleans, Library of Congress; Dr. and Mrs. Eugene A. Stead, Jr., Duke University Medical Center, Durham, N.C.; Myron E. Wegman, M.D., University of Michigan, Ann Arbor.

politics, black, white, and Chinese. I will undoubtedly miss some, but even a partial listing is a reminder that the exchanges are essentially a one-way street; there have now been twelve Chinese physicians here and seventy-five American physicians there:

Harold Aaron, M.D.	John K. Koo, M.D.
Herbert Abrams, M.D.	Matthew H. M. Lee, M.D.
Harry Becker, M.D.	Chen-pien Li, M.D.
Thelma Blackman, M.D.	John Chan Nao Liu, M.D.
Freeman Cary, M.D.	Paul Lowinger, M.D.
Melvin A. Casberg, M.D.	Bernard Lown, M.D.
Edmund Casey, M.D.	Abraham T. Lu, M.D.
Ralph J. Cazort, M.D.	Frank McDowell, M.D.
James Y. P. Chen, M.D.	Ronald A. Malt, M.D.
Tsung O. Cheng, M.D.	Marion Mann, M.D.
David T. Chi, M.D.	R. J. Pearson, M.D.
Montague W. Cobb, M.D.	Alfred Peng, M.D.
E. Leon Cooper, M.D.	Constance S. Pittman, M.D.
Eliot Corday, M.D.	Samuel Rosen, M.D.
Michael E. DeBakey, M.D.	Abraham Rudolph, M.D.
E. Grey Dimond, M.D.	Ernest Saward, M.D.
Donald B. Effler, M.D.	Alex Shulman, M.D.
Effie O. Ellis, M.D.	Victor Sidel, M.D.
Y. C. Fung, M.D.	Calvin H. Sinnette, M.D.
H. Jack Geiger, M.D.	Mitchell Spellman, M.D.
Jeoffrey Gordon, M.D.	Benjamin Spock, M.D.
Richard P. Green, M.D., R. Ph.	David A. Stadtner, M.D.
Chih-tang Han, M.D.	H. J. C. Swan, M.D.
Wayne Y. Ho, M.D.	Paul Teng, M.D.
Frederick Holschuh, M.D.	Walter Tkach, M.D.
Hsi-fan Hsu, M.D.	Andrew L. Thomas, M.D.
Joseph Jen-yuan Hsu, M.D.	George Tolbert, M.D.
Frederick F. Kao, M.D.	Sanford Sui Tom, M.D.
Arnold M. Katz, M.D.	Emerson Walden, M.D.
Suzanne B. Knoebel, M.D.	Chi-Tang Wen, M.D.
Helen Yen Koo, M.D.	Jerry David Wu, M.D.

Chapter Thirteen

THE NEW LOOK OF
CHINESE MEDICINE

OTHER EVIDENCE of the return to a stable level of operation of medicine and science after the Cultural Revolution is the re-appearance of the *Chinese Medical Journal.* This journal, the national medical journal comparable to our *Journal of the American Medical Association,* was suspended from publication in 1966. Cross-communication between medical workers and investigators within China essentially stopped for a six-year period. In fact, at the time of our first trip to Peking, in September, 1971, the Chinese Medical Association was operating with but a skeleton staff and was primarily a vehicle for handling arrangements for foreign visiting physicians. Contrary to our American academic aphorism "Publish or perish," it quickly became obvious that in new China, at least during the height of the Cultural Revolution, publishing *and* perishing might be one and the same activity.

The appearance of the first medical journal is good evidence that the Chinese medical system has recovered from the Cultural Revolution. The journal, in Chinese of course, is brightly covered in green, contains good and thorough scientific data, black-and-white and color photographs, and—an especially important fact—English and only English summaries. The editor, Dr. Weng Yun-chin, is an excellent man, a physician who speaks English and has had considerable editorial experience. Considering the narrow guidelines through which he must thread his editorial policy, he indeed has a difficult task. The *Journal* appeared in January, 1973, and is available monthly by direct mail from Peking to the United States. Subscription can be made through: Guozi Shudian, P.O. Box 399, Peking, China.

The articles have been interesting from the viewpoint of both subject matter and authorship. As evidence of the hesitation created by the Cultural Revolution, many of the articles indicate only the institution but not the author. The subject matter is impressive and is an exciting hint of the exotic potential of combining the scientific accuracy of Western medicine and the unknown possibilities of Chinese traditional medicine. From the first six issues, I have taken some article headings to give an indication of subject matter and origin of the work. (The enumeration is mine.)

1. "Replantation of Severed Limbs and Fingers." Research Laboratory for Replantation of Severed Limbs, Shanghai Sixth People's Hospital, Shanghai. *CMJ*, no. 1 (January, 1973), p. 1.
2. "Acute Myocardial Infarction Treated with Traditional and Western Medicine." Hua Shan Hospital, Shanghai First Medical College, Shanghai. *CMJ*, no. 1 (January, 1973), p. 7.
3. "Combined Traditional and Western Medicine in Acute Abdominal Conditions." Nan K'ai Hospital, Tientsin. *CMJ*, no. 1 (January, 1973), p. 8.
4. "Acupuncture Anesthesia in Neurosurgery." Department of Anesthesiology, Hsuan Wu Hospital, Peking. *CMJ*, no. 2 (February, 1973), p. 15.
5. "Acupuncture Anesthesia in Thyroidectomy." Shanghai First People's Hospital, Shanghai. *CMJ*, no. 2 (February, 1973), p. 17.
6. "Laryngectomy under Acupuncture Anesthesia." Eye, Ear, Nose and Throat Hospital of Shanghai First Medical College, Shanghai. *CMJ*, no. 2 (February, 1973), p. 18.
7. "Pulmonary Resections under Acupuncture Anesthesia." Shanghai First Tuberculosis Hospital, Shanghai. *CMJ*, no. 2 (February, 1973), p. 19.
8. "Acupuncture Anesthesia in Thoracic Surgery: Clinical Analysis of 818 Cases." Section of Thoracic Surgery of Peking Acupuncture Anesthesia Co-ordinating Group. *CMJ*, no. 2 (February, 1973), p. 20.

9. "Acupuncture Anesthesia in Cardiac Surgery." Thoracic Section, Acupuncture Anesthesia Group of Second Teaching Hospital of Hunan Medical College, Changsha, Hunan. *CMJ*, no. 2 (February, 1973), p. 21.

10. "Acupuncture Anesthesia in Splenectomy: Report of 305 Cases." Ch'angshan County People's Hospital, Ch'angshan, Chekiang. *CMJ*, no. 2 (February, 1973), p. 22.

11. "Acupuncture Anesthesia in Pediatric Surgery: Report of 1,308 Cases." Department of Surgery, Peking Children's Hospital, Peking. *CMJ*, no. 2 (February, 1973), p. 23.

12. "Acupuncture Anesthesia for Operations in Shock and Critical Cases." Department of Anesthesiology, Teaching Hospital of Anhwei Medical College, Hofei, Anhwei. *CMJ*, no. 2 (February, 1973), p. 24.

13. "Effect of Needling of the Philtrum on Hemorrhagic Shock in Cats." Department of Physiology, Anhwei Medical College, Hofei, Anhwei. *CMJ*, no. 2 (February, 1973), p. 25.

14. "Traditional-Western Medicine in Treatment of Infantile Pneumonia." Department of Pediatrics, Peking Friendship Hospital, Peking. *CMJ*, no. 2 (February, 1973), p. 30.

15. "Electrical Response to Nocuous Stimulation and Its Inhibition in Nucleus Centralis Lateralis of Thalamus in Rabbits." Shanghai Institute of Physiology, Shanghai. *CMJ*, no. 3 (March, 1973), p. 31.

16. "The Role of Midbrain Reticular Formation in Acupuncture Anesthesia." Acupuncture Anesthesia Co-ordinating Group of Shanghai College of Traditional Chinese Medicine, Shanghai Normal College and Shu Kuang Hospital of Shanghai College of Traditional Chinese Medicine, Shanghai. *CMJ*, no. 3 (March, 1973), p. 32.

17. "Electrophysiologic Study of Spinal Reflexes under Acupuncture Anesthesia." Acupuncture Anesthesia Research Unit, Hsu Yi County People's Hospital, Hsu Yi County, Kiangsu. *CMJ*, no. 3 (March, 1973), p. 33.

18. "Preliminary Experimental Morphologic and Electron Microscopic Studies of the Connection between Acupuncture Points on the Limbs and the Segments of the Spinal Cord." Morphologic Section of the Acupuncture Anesthesia Re-

search Unit, Shenyang Medical College, Shenyang. *CMJ*, no. 3 (March, 1973), p. 34.

19. "Effect of Acupuncture on Pain Threshold of Human Skin." Research Group of Acupuncture Anesthesia, Peking Medical College, Peking. *CMJ*, no. 3 (March, 1973), p. 35.

20. "Pharmaceutical Studies of a Traditional Antidiphtheria Mixture." Antidiptheria Mixture Research Group, Institute of Chinese Materia Medica, Academy of Traditional Chinese Medicine, Peking. *CMJ*, no. 3 (March, 1973), p. 39.

21. "Clinical Application of *Ilex chinensis* Sims in Treatment of Burns." Burn Unit, Teaching Hospital of Nantung Medical College, Nantung. *CMJ*, no. 4 (April, 1973), p. 48.

22. "Clinical Observations on Action of Ointment Yuchuang No. 10 in Separation of Eschars." Burn Unit, Jiu Chin Hospital of Shanghai Second Medical College and Shanghai Third Traditional Chinese Pharmaceutical Factory, Shanghai. *CMJ*, no. 4 (April, 1973), p. 51.

23. "The Metabolic Fate of Securinine." Institute of Materia Medica, Chinese Academy of Medical Sciences, Peking. *CMJ*, no. 4 (April, 1973), p. 52.

24. "Anisodamine Therapy of Diseases of Acute Microcirculatory Disturbances." Department of Pediatrics, Peking Friendship Hospital; Department of Pharmacology, Institute of Materia Medica, Chinese Academy of Medical Sciences; and First Laboratory of an Institute of Chinese Academy of Medical Sciences. *CMJ*, no. 5 (May, 1973), p. 55.

25. "Combined Traditional and Western Medicine in Treatment of Tuberculous Cystospasm: Report of 4 Cases." Departments of Urology, Peking Friendship Hospital and Kuang An Men Hospital of the Academy of Traditional Chinese Medicine, Peking. *CMJ*, no. 5 (May, 1973), p. 65.

26. "Replantation of Severed Limbs: Analysis of 40 Cases." Department of Traumatology and Orthopedics, Peking Chishueit'an Hospital, Peking. *CMJ*, no. 6 (June, 1973), p. 67.

27. "Experience in Replantation of Severed Fingers." Department of Surgery, First Teaching Hospital of Chung Shan Medical College, Kwangchow. *CMJ*, no. 6 (June, 1973), p. 71.

28. "Replantation of Limbs after Resection of Neoplastic Segment: Report of 8 Cases." Research Laboratory for Replantation of Severed Limbs, Shanghai Sixth People's Hospital, Shanghai. *CMJ*, no. 6 (June, 1973), p. 72.

The intense interest and new level of success in replantation of fingers, arms, hands, feet, and legs is reflected in Articles 1, 26 27, and 28. The wide experience in the clinical use of acupuncture anesthesia throughout China and in all fields of surgery can be noted in Articles 4, 5, 6, 7, 8, 9, 10, 11, and 12. Articles 12, 13, 15, 16, 17, 18, and 19 give a rationale for the analgesia produced by needling. The attempt to make pharmacological sense from the almost witch's brew of traditional medicines begins to be defined in the work reported in Articles 2, 3, 14, 20, 21, 22, 23 24, and 25. The unusual scope of *all* of these articles must make other medical research workers aware that, right or wrong, the Chinese are taking a new approach. The reports are at such a tangent from Western medical research that initially we will be inclined to disregard or downgrade them. However, a moment of thoughtful reflection must remind us that the Chinese, government and investigator, are not only very capable but also very unlikely to place in the medical literature anything which is not accurate. The Chinese are proud and sensitive; the appearance of the new *Journal* and these very carefully selected articles is deliberate notice to the professional world of new Chinese research.

One objective in citing these articles is to convey the information that the Chinese scientifically trained physicians and basic scientists are well on their way to seeking an understanding of the possible principles behind acupuncture. These scientists are just as curious as any Westerner and have had to overcome their major professional reservations about acupuncture. Their willingness now to apply scientific methods and their close working relationships with the traditional physician should give the Chinese a considerable success in this field. One hopes the West will give the closest of attention to the Chinese reports and will not be turned away by the occasional burst of Marxism. From the new *Chinese Medical Journal*, I have placed in the Appendix two complete English abstracts, not only for their information value, as I realize most readers are not physicians, but to give two clear examples of the unique potential of current Chinese research work.

The one abstract demonstrates the complete mixture of basic science, modern therapeutics, and ancient acupuncture sites, all being brought to bear on the question of "How does acupuncture anesthesia work?" The other abstract equally utilizes the best of modern physiology and modern surgery in the replacement of limbs.

In contradistinction to these well-done research studies, I have seen other variations of acupuncture and herb usage which I cannot rationalize on a scientific basis.

First, and by the millions of treatments per day, is the uncritical, almost dart-board approach going on at every level. Acupuncture is taught in grade school and in factories, and is the national first line of therapeutic defense. The whole ancient practice of pulse feeling, herb dispensing, acupuncturing is going on, not only as it has for thousands of years but with a considerable upsurge because of Mao's urgings. During the long years of Western missionary medicine, Chinese traditional medicine was essentially black-market medicine or poor-people medicine. In the cities and universities where the missionary influence was maximal, Chinese traditional medicine was banned, and such subjects were not permitted in the teaching hospitals or in the classroom. This interdiction had little effect on the rural peasant. He did not have the benefit of Western medicine, and therefore the concepts of Chinese traditional medicine stayed alive, beyond the missionaries' influence.

Much of what I would describe as wholesale acupuncture is disturbing to a Western observer. The lack of training and the risk of hepatitis from unclean needles is distressing. The rationale which must be accepted, however, is that this is at least a reasonably safe procedure to offer as the first line of psychosomatic support to the world's largest medical practice. Perhaps the needles are not free of hepatitis antigen, but also they're not acting as conduits for unneeded and potentially harmful vitamins, hormones, steroids, and expensive mixtures.

One can only accept the fact that acupuncture and herbs are emotionally acceptable to the Chinese, and the nationwide non-critical use is in part psychosomatic, certainly economical, and at worst not causing much harm. I have seen acupuncture in several dozen situations where I could not believe that the needle was adequately prepared or that the manipulator had any awareness of disease transmission. Children in the fifth grade in Shanghai were busily acupuncturing each other, complete with manikins for study. In the factory health station, in the hotel, in the commune brigade health station, on the train, in the deaf-mute school, all about and everywhere, one sees acupuncture used as therapy. The list of reasons for the use of acupuncture was usually reassuring, however. Problems of muscle ache, strain, spasm, of backache, stiff neck, all have a least a muscular basis, and such needling may well be therapeutic.

An example of the wholesale use of acupuncture was in the physiotherapy department of a large hospital in Wuhan. Three middle-aged ladies were seated, busily knitting and chatting, each with acupuncture needles in her ears. Each was being treated for tiredness, weakness, and malaise specifically labeled by the attending doctor as "neurasthenia." Doctors' offices throughout the world have similar middle-aged ladies, but I had not seen such skillful group therapy—and economical, benign therapy. The needles were placed quickly, in a matter of seconds, by the doctor, and he was free to see other patients for the remainder of the thirty-minute treatment. At the end of the session, the needles were removed by an attendant and the three ladies left together, spirits improved and at least not burdened with vitamin B_{12}, or E, or B_6.

I found no claims for acupuncture in the treatment of cancer and leukemia. The Chinese approach to the cancer problem of Edgar Snow and the acute appendicitis of James Reston was exactly like ours. In Snow's circumstance, there was the same set of alternatives one would find in any advanced country: surgery, X-ray, or chemotherapy. The Chinese did turn to an herbal remedy in the hope of improving his nutrition and his ability to perhaps tolerate chemotherapy. In Reston's case, he was introduced into the mysteries of China when, after surgery, his severe "gas colic" was treated by acupuncture. Mr. Reston's appendicitis was treated surgically; however, in both Canton and Wuhan I heard detailed discussion of an herbal decoction, taken by mouth, which is said to stop acute appendicitis in 90 percent of those receiving it. In various institutions, I saw patients who were under treatment for well-recognized problems (using Western medical terms) and the treatment was herbal. The Western science worker is not going to be comfortable with much of this pragmatic clinical testing of herbal medicines. However, in the present Chinese political setting, a factor that must be considered, some of the work is excellent, and repeatedly there was evidence of herbs with active ingredients of clinical promise. For example, at the Fu Wai Hospital, serious therapeutic studies are under way in cardiogenic shock, angina pectoris, and hypertension. In Wuhan, herbal treatment of pneumococcal pneumonia, neisserian meningitis, and cystitis was under study, comparing herbal results to that obtained with our usual antibiotics. Some of these results have already appeared in the first issues of the *Chinese Medical Journal.*

Should the United States be doing more in terms of cooperative efforts in research with China? Such efforts will come very slowly. My own reasons for involvement have been, at all points, to bring the West and China into a livable understanding, not only in medicine. Medicine is an area in which useful altruistic exploration can occur, but that may not be sufficient reason for much change on the part of the Chinese. The deep sense of hurt and alienation following not only our attitude of the past twenty-five years, but the one hundred years of humiliation at the hands of the West will not be overcome by the enthusiasm of a handful of American visitors. In fact, medicine may not be the best avenue for relationships. A more pragmatic need by the United States to balance its budget and for the Chinese to obtain wheat may bring an economic relationship. The likelihood of large personal exchanges seems remote at this time. Some will continue, carefully spaced, but China will stand apart, clearly independent. Dr. Jerome Frank, speaking before a Senate hearing of Senator Fulbright's, said, "The first and probably most difficult step is psychological. We must re-examine the image we have formed about China . . . bearing in mind from a historical viewpoint the humiliation it has suffered. Undoubtedly, we must be prepared to go further and to accept from them a kind of symbolic humiliation."

The July, 1973, issue of the *Chinese Medical Journal* had thirteen major articles. Eleven of these were typical, well-done, medical science literature reports. However, in the position reserved in most medical journals for the premier presentation, there were two articles bearing the titles "Chairman Mao's Poem Consolidates Victory over Schistosomiasis" and "Chairman Mao's Health Line Inspires a District." The first article carried, among others, this paragraph:

First, coordinating the study of works of Marx, Engels, Lenin, Stalin and Chairman Mao's works with the movement to criticize revisionism and rectify the style of work, maintaining vigilance against sabotage by political enemies, deepening health consciousness, and consolidating the results of antischistosomiasis work . . . they carried out their tasks.

This, translated into action, means that through Party leadership, everyone was organized, worked together, and took the necessary public health measures to decrease snail population, examine peasants, and institute treatment. The quoted paragraph is a good example of the phrases used regularly throughout "official" China.

Chapter Fourteen

THE PEKING ACUPUNCTURE
ANESTHESIA
CO-ORDINATING GROUP

༓༓༓༓

IN 1973, I had the advantage of a third trip to China, a lengthy one in the spring. My collection of information was further aided by the intense three-week experience in the United States when I accompanied the Chinese physicians. My declared interest in fostering American research efforts into all aspects of Chinese medicine has brought me into contact with a remarkable array of interested American investigators, varying from recognized accurate workers to well-meaning but painfully non-critical enthusiasts.

The future prospects for finding new therapeutic products from the unbelievable array of Chinese herbs and remedies is good. Such analytical work is time-consuming and expensive, but eventually active ingredients will be identified and therapeutic trials accomplished. The Chinese are likely to obtain such information faster than our own superb materia medica and pharmacology teams. The reasons for this are several, but first and most important is the fact that the Chinese scientist is emotionally prepared to believe that such ancient remedies as Tibetan red flower and dragon tooth root are therapeutic and therefore are worth the effort of scientific study. The Chinese scientist is emotionally prepared because he lives and breathes in a civilization that has for several thousand years placed its faith in these agents. He also is emotionally prepared because he lives today in a society that is encouraged through every possible form of propaganda to believe that correct Communist thought is the same as correct scientific thought which is the same as correct

Chairman Mao thought. Indoctrination is a part of life in today's China, and one of the principal barriers to the possible advantages of scientific cooperation between our two countries is the burden the Chinese scientist bears in that he must somehow credit Mao Tse-tung Thought with any scientific progress.

For Americans, this political sloganeering mixed into scientific reporting produces documents whose basic accuracy seems suspect. If, however, one can train himself to ignore these Mao tributes as but the toll the Chinese scientists must pay to cross the scientific literature bridge, then the real merit of the basic work is impressive. One might remind himself of the American requirement that the elected American official begins his journey by swearing upon the Bible—but his route thereafter certainly takes some major detours..

In 1972, there appeared a statement in English prepared by the Peking Acupuncture Anesthesia Co-ordinating Group entitled "Acupuncture Anesthesia: A Brief Introduction." This was sent to me by the group and represents the first major effort to extend information on acupuncture anesthesia to the United States. The hour-long movie made by this group was shown in Kansas City and is available there to anyone wishing to see it. I am printing their statement in the Appendix in its entirety because of the unique nature of the information and, secondarily, to give the reader an example of how the scientific message is woven around necessary political slogans.

The opening paragraph is one to make the American research worker wince, and is an example of why real scholarly exchanges between the two countries will be difficult and limited:

Our country's medical and scientific workers at large under the guidance of Chairman Mao's revolutionary line in health work respond enthusiastically to Chairman Mao's great call, "Chinese medicine and pharmacology are a great treasure-house; efforts should be made to explore them and raise them to a higher level." By combining revolutionary zeal with scientific spirit, applying modern scientific knowledge and methods, they have summed up and improved on the experiences of time-honored traditional Chinese medicine in stopping pain and curing ailments with needling. After many years of repeated studies, they have succeeded in creating China's unique anesthetic technic—acupuncture anesthesia.

This report from the Peking Acupuncture team is a substantial medical document. The reader can easily sift out the compliments to correct political orientation and to ancestral medicine —and find accurate descriptions of the necessary clinical technique of needle manipulation to produce anesthesia adequate for major surgery. The earnest desire to communicate with peer professionals comes through to the reader. The role of electrical stimulation is defined. Short of a trip to China, this Peking report is an effective introduction to anesthesia without drugs and documents well the reasons why Edgar Snow and, subsequently, I myself knew there was a physiological, not political, truth in what we had seen.

The Peking Acupuncture Anesthesia Co-ordinating Group is but one of several cooperative teams in China working hard to develop both the clinical use and a basic scientific explanation for acupuncture. The first truly Sino-American cooperative effort in acupuncture therapy is under way, with Samuel and Helen Rosen trying acupuncture as therapy for deafness, with careful audiographic control, in both Peking and New York City.

It is apparent from reading the report of the Coordinating Group and from review of the new *Chinese Medical Journal* that the Chinese have come upon a means of increasing a person's ability to endure pain. I use this phrase because it seems apparent that the signal does begin at the pained part of the body but in its transit is attenuated and can be tolerated or ignored.

The question of acupuncture is at last being looked at with an open mind. The only reasonable approach is one of asking why, of being hopeful that there is truth in it, and accepting the facts, one way or the other.

A subsequent group of Chinese scientists came to the United States in November, 1973, with special interests in the physiology of pain and biomedical engineering. This eight-person group toured widely and visited medical research units throughout the United States. In basic discussions on explanations for acupuncture anesthesia, the matter was thoroughly explored. A substantial document, *The Proceedings of the National Institute of Health Acupuncture Research Conference* (February 28–March 1, 1973), has appeared. Reputable universities are offering seminars on American Acupuncture!

American acupuncture falls into two unequal categories. The vast majority seems to be, just as one would have feared, a clutter of uncritical, money-making quackupuncture.

The United States has more than its share of semi-neurotic, complaining, worrying, underused, and overstressed healthy people. I say healthy people because most of us are never free of some ache, pain, tremble, quiver, or start. Most of us have a little backache, a little stomach upset, a little headache, a night of wakefulness. Living is not just one glorious burst of well-being but is essentially a matter of being involved in responsibility sufficient to make us forget the sputterings of the human engine. Acupuncture has provided a safe, simple additional, non-bottled solace for these people. I do not really object to this form of psychosomatic care, and, from observation, suspect that much of the role of acupuncture in China, now and through history, has been similar.

There is a more significant category, now still small in volume but, I believe, destined to be the larger contribution to mankind. That is acupuncture for the relief of pain, the remission of spasm, the breaking of a pain cycle, the interruption of a "trigger" point that has disabled the patient. The use of acupuncture in this area will lead in many directions, including the simple needling for wryneck, for nerve pain after injury (whether caused by bullet, lumbar disc, auto accident, or cancer), on to electrical stimulation of major nerves and the spinal cord to make endurable the incessant terrible burning nerve pain described as causalgia.

American physicians were already using many of the techniques of acupuncture, sometimes unknowingly. Janet Travell, physician to President John Kennedy, gained his confidence of her professional skills by relieving his back pain, after several back operations had not helped. Part of what she did was to inject by needle a local anesthetic into "trigger areas." The recognition of trigger areas and subsequent muscle spasm and their total relief by needling was a true contribution by Dr. Travell and, one must say, a contribution not well appreciated by her colleagues because they could not explain her theory with their own accepted anatomical rules. Acupuncture today, as it will be used by the American physician, is in part exactly what Janet Travell tried to offer to her colleagues more than twenty-five years ago. I have had in my own files for more than twenty years articles written by her on the subject of "trigger zones," and in one of those she made the bland, uncluttered comment that she had found that the insertion of the needle *without* the injection of a local anesthetic often resulted in complete relief of pain! I have not seen Janet for several years, but I hope she is enjoying this latter-day, oriental verification of her life's work.

Another American physician also came upon similar therapeutic success, although by a different route. Dr. C. N. Shealy of Wisconsin, as early as 1967, successfully relieved intractable pain from cancer by implanting electrodes adjacent to the spinal column and electrically stimulating the nerve pathway for pain. The needle at the skin of Chinese acupuncture (and Janet Travell) and the larger surgical concept of implanted electrical stimulators of Shealy are all part of the same story. Modern medical science, modern medical schools, and modern medical practice now have new techniques of treatment, new results to explain scientifically—and considerable embarrassment at their persistent unwillingness to take an honest look at an old-new idea.

We Americans may be late in discovering a subject, but when we do, we take it up with enthusiasm.

Chapter Fifteen

A SOCIETY WITHOUT NARCOTICS
AND VENEREAL DISEASE

To ANALYZE one of the most formidable accomplishments in the health care field in China since 1949, let us ask ourselves what has happened to the general public health in the United States in that same period of time. As a framework for discussion, compare two major problems which involve the large area of social medicine. In using the phrase "social medicine," I am referring to those diseases or problems which seem to have a relationship to society as a whole rather than to an individual and his disease.

Let us consider narcotics and venereal disease.

These are critical social issues, because in addition to the effect on the individual, there are other factors which involve the family, disease spread, crime, and prostitution. Our American society has not found a solution; the Chinese have eliminated these problems.

In substantial conversations with Ma Hai-teh and other physicians in China, I have begun to understand how these areas have been handled. I cannot claim to understand how similar solutions could occur in the United States. The accomplishments of the Chinese in the resolution of these areas require a complex of factors, some of which do not fit the American scene.

Among these factors was a straightforward public policy announcing that there would be no further use of narcotics, except medically. Such an announcement has no merit unless the public essentially endorses it, as we learned from our own attempt at prohibition.

The Chinese government obtained the public's attention by massive use of all education media. Hour by hour, day in and day out, the radio was used to educate. Newspapers and posters were used as education vehicles. The clear public policy of absolutely no further narcotics to be tolerated within China was given a specific cut-off date and was reinforced by constant newspaper and radio coverage. More important was the skilled Party membership, which represents the direct arm of the government and which has a direct personal contact with every neighborhood, every household, every work team. These men and women, the cadres, had learned to work together at Yenan over an eleven-year period (which length of time many of us forget); the Communist management system was seasoned. The absolutely personal and invasive role of these Party representatives can be appreciated by listing their tasks, as Jan Myrdal has done.*

The tasks of a Communist party group at the village level are described:

1) To organize women to take an active part in production;
2) To spread literacy among women and get them to study and take an interest in social questions;
3) To help them do their domestic work effectively and economically, to help them when any economic problem arises in their family;
4) To teach them personal and public hygiene; and
5) To give help and advice over marriage or other personal problems of wedded life.

In February, 1950, Chou En-lai issued a directive forbidding growing, manufacturing, selling, or using opium. It was an "honest directive, one which was sincerely meant," to quote Ma Hai-teh. Anyone selling narcotics would be arrested. If, after such persuasion, the offender continued to sell narcotics, he was subject to being shot. Ma Hai-teh had not seen an execution, but had read of them in the Canton area. Anyone addicted to narcotics would be helped to free himself and would have employment. The essential technique of stopping the drug was that of abrupt, total stopping. Occasionally, a decreasing amount over a two-week period was the route followed, but usually complete and sudden stopping was practiced. Other medications were very rarely substituted, in fact, they had no such drugs. Magnesium sulfate by injection was almost the only sedative. During this

* Jan Myrdal, *Report from a Chinese Village* (New York: New American Library, 1966), p. 255.

entire period, intense education was carried on, which, in part, consisted in telling the individual that it was not his fault that he had used narcotics, but that it was the fault of the old society, which had done this to him.

Group discussions, guided by cadres, were carried on constantly. The entire country mobilized itself to wipe out narcotics, immediately.

The Chinese approach to these massive health drives has been to *politicize* the issue. Instead of delegating the specific health problem to the health departments or to the individual doctor or community hospital, as we have done, for example, with alcoholism, the Chinese government made the problem a national issue related to patriotism, citizenship, and duty to the country. The elimination of venereal disease was a declared policy of the Communist Party, and therefore there was no debate or individual latitude. The straightforward message was that good citizens do not have venereal disease.

This technique was referred to by Ma Hai-teh as the "mass line," in which every single citizen is involved; intense propaganda efforts, continuous group discussions led by trained leaders, the mobilization of all social organizations from youth league to neighborhood group, have been the fundamental educational plan for every major health campaign. This, for instance, includes the campaigns to eliminate flies, mosquitoes, sparrows, and rats, the anti–venereal disease campaign, the hygiene drives to clean up homes, to collect feces correctly, to carry out physical fitness programs.

Why does such a program work in China? In narcotic containment, one major fact which distinguishes the ability of the Chinese to carry out a prohibition was the closure of the borders to illegal narcotic entry. Our image of the remoteness of China makes this seem feasible, but the vast rugged southern border of China adjacent to Burma is near the source of much of the world's opium, and if there had been a market in, say, Canton or Shanghai, one assumes that the narcotics would have got there. The absolute ruling that the seller of narcotics was an enemy of the people and subject to death was undoubtedly the major reason why narcotics no longer arrived in the cities. The other fact of

Chinese life, that no citizen may move more than a certain number of miles from his place of residence without a permit, obviously limits drug movement. This total lack of mobility would certainly have a major effect if instituted in the United States!

Still, Ma Hai-teh made clear to me that it was not police action that stopped narcotics totally and almost instantly. He attributes the result to the massive "mass line" public education, plus the remarkable willingness of the Chinese to be recognized as good citizens. All factors, he believes, were necessary: (a) an unwavering, non-negotiable policy, not subject to debate, that all drug usage must stop by a defined date, (b) the policy that the user was guilty of no crime but was a victim of a bad previous social system and would be helped to full rehabilitation without stigma, (c) the line that selling was a crime against the people, punishable by death, (d) the mobilization of every form of propaganda and education, building up to an intense (e) mass awareness and enthusiasm of the entire population, and (f) neighborhood and family penetration by skilled representatives of the Party.

The same sequence was followed in the elimination of venereal disease and prostitution.* A date for the end was declared, all houses were closed, and rehabilitation programs were begun, frequently on the premises. Venereal disease and other health problems were treated. Medication was free. Education for new careers was begun. Many prostitutes become nurses. Many were resettled into new jobs and factories or returned to their families in the countryside. Again, it was the firm propaganda theme that they were prostitutes because they had been misused by the previous bad social system. They were told they were now citizens of a new China and they could start fresh again. Many of the girls stayed in the house, which was reopened as a small shop, and they became seamstresses or developed a handicraft. Even the procurers were given an opportunity at rehabilitation, but if the procurer was an especially evil person and had been wantonly cruel, then trial and condemnation did occur.

* See Appendix D. Quotation from Joshua S. Horn, *Away with All Pests* (New York: Monthly Review Press, 1969). Dr. Horn, an English physician, was in China at the time of these large "mass line" movements.

As Mai Hai-teh told me of these vast social actions, I found myself still uncomprehending. My lifetime as a member of a society in which there is such remarkable individual expression, in which civil liberty is real, in which easy movement through city, state, and nation is expected, makes me unable to re-create the Chinese setting. It is only if I introduce a different form of government or a remarkable moral renaissance to my thinking that I am able to understand how the elimination of narcotics, venereal disease, and crime could be brought about in the United States. The additional quality that has been captured in the Chinese social revolution is that the Chinese have developed individual and personal pride in what has been done by new China. This sense of pride in being Chinese has been multiplied by calling forth the good qualities of human nature and by instituting a national educational program stressing the importance of good personal conduct. The strong government policy called Mao Tse-tung Thought sets the guidelines, but through remarkably skilled persuasion and "mass line" effort, Mao Tse-tung Thought has become a vast philosophical code of conduct. The punitive and coercive arm is also there, but in recent years it has been lightly used.

Through a series of nationwide exhortations, most of China's social diseases and infectious diseases were wiped out by the early 1960s. In addition to venereal diseases, narcotics, and prostitution, other mass line health efforts invaded the entire spectrum of Chinese life. Homosexuality was equally defined as an unacceptable social pattern.

The very basic issues of nourishment were solved by improved farming techniques and water reservoirs. The entire country was damaged from the years of war. Peace itself was therapeutic. Fields were tilled, irrigation mended, livestock established. Immense numbers of physical laborers, both volunteer and "persuaded," built bridges, dams, and canals. The ancient and essential use of human excreta for fertilizer was formalized and cement privies built. Methods of sealing the night soil to cause heat generation and the death of parasites became national policy carried forward by the cadres. The need for this essential waste material in maintaining a living, productive earth is also a lesson to be learned by the West. Our remarkable enthusiasm for sanitation has essentially been based on the total removal or destruction of waste from foodstuffs which came from the earth and were processed through the human body. Our interruption of the cycle which would return this material to the earth has been partly met by creating chemical fertilizers. These new chemical fertilizers aggravate man's race for survival by generating pollution in their production and permanently destroying their original earth source—for example, natural gas. The West now, almost as a national emergency, must remove the emotional barricade which makes such a thought repugnant and unclean and define methods for returning human fertilizer to the soil.

Massive educational programs on why water must be boiled, why flies must be killed, also became vehicles for the cadre to carry out along with other policies of communization. Mass assaults on mosquitoes, flies, sparrows, and rats brought entire cities into action at the same time, and high public excitement was created by comparing neighborhood against neighborhood for diligence, and in encouraging success as part of the national defense. *Health and patriotism became paired words.* To use Ma Hai-teh's words, health was politicized.

Chapter Sixteen

THE CALMING OF PASSIONS

THE REPORTS from all visitors to China seem adequately uniform to confirm the success of the Chinese health system in terms of problems which could be called "public health." The cleaning up of canals, irrigation ditches, gutters, ponds, rivers, courtyards, and houses is not exactly medical care as we think of it in the West, but such measures were an essential first step in getting vermin, lice, and disease-spreading pests under control. The absence of litter is a frequent comment of the visitor, but the purpose of this massive cleaning up of the debris and garbage of centuries was a major health effort; the aesthetic result was a secondary benefit. The war in Korea had been a useful ally in a sense to the Chinese government in this massive clean-up campaign. Warning of impending biological warfare by the United States, whether fact or fiction, was a prime message distributed by the Chinese authorities. The general population was urged to eliminate animals who might be infected and to get rid of stagnant ponds and sources of fecal contamination, as means of improving their protection in case of biological and bacteriological war.

Scrawny village dogs were a familiar feature of old China. Their fleas, worms, and kala azar were a target of the new public health approach, and one rarely sees a dog in today's China. I have seen two, in fact, one a family pet in the home of Dr. Hans Müller and the other a puppy belonging to the caretaker of a museum in Sian.

The use of boiled water and the mass line assault on venereal disease, leprosy, ringworm, malaria, and tuberculosis have either eliminated these diseases or contained them. Schistosomiasis has been materially decreased and new cases found quickly and treated. The canal and irrigation nature of much of the farming of south China has made this disease an especially difficult one to control. The public has learned of the role of the snail, the symptoms of the disease, and the need for treatment. Snail gathering and snail killing have had the mass line approach.

Adequate food has eliminated one of the greatest scourges of old China, famine and starvation. Good nourishment has stopped rickets, and deformed bodies from rickets, poliomyelitis, tuberculosis, and osteomyelitis are very rarely seen.

Spraying, de-bugging, vaccination, boiled water, better handling of night soil, elimination of pest reservoirs, good midwifery have stopped plagues, epidemics, and infant and mother mortality.

All these things have been done, and the health system today has permitted the development of a gigantic population of straight, strong bodies with good white, even teeth. The Chinese woman's foot is no longer bound, she walks with a long, determined stride and is fully employed in the fields, factories, and army. In the health professions, she makes up half of the new classes. The Chinese woman is liberated—and out of the home, hard at work.

What problem perhaps have resulted? Are all things good? What are the bad health facts? Or, stated differently, have the past twenty-four years seen any adverse changes in the health challenges in China?

The obvious challenge is the race between sufficient food and increasing population. The Chinese have successfully generated enough new yield from their land to keep ahead of their population growth. The buying of wheat from the United States and Canada is perhaps not as large a warning signal of impending food shortage as one might initially think. China has consistently sold rice during these years and for a better price per bushel than the cost for the imported wheat. Further, the Chinese have used rice as a method of overseas aid and trade. Chinese rice goes to Ceylon (Sri Lanka) in exchange for rubber.

Still, the improved health of the Chinese population, combined with the numbers, can only be a combination which could explode the population. The health care system is active with major efforts to decrease the incidence of birth. Barefoot doctors, factory health workers, are vigorously using the techniques of persuasion and mass line action to convince the Chinese that a "two baby family" is ideal. All usual forms of birth control are available and officially sanctioned. One additional factor, and again an example of the large influence of public opinion on Chinese behavior, has been the general acceptance of celibacy before marriage and the postponement of marriage until the mid- to late twenties. The removal of these fertile years from baby production mathematically decreases by more than a third the childbearing years of an entire nation.

The Western visitor has difficulty in accepting the fact of national celibacy. Again, the constancy of the reports from a variety of reputable observers cannot be disregarded. Our own daily life is a continual barrage of boy-girl, man-woman, he-she, him-her situations. Reminders of sex are built into our entire environment. Expressive behavior is urged by our psychologists. We have encouraged ourselves to believe that all of this leads to being "well adjusted" and that such behavior patterns (I am including the entire range of sex activity, in all of its enthusiasm) are the expected, normal manifestations of maturity in a liberated society. The Chinese have rejected all of this, and instead have defined rules of modesty, celibacy, and non-sexual expression in dress and deed.

I conclude this chapter on public health by suggesting that the Chinese non-sex program perhaps has wholesome public health significance. Instead of the pent-up hormonal and emotional storms which we ourselves assume must happen if sex expression is not permitted—in fact, encouraged—the Chinese seem freed, calm, and serene. Western psychologists and behaviorists cannot disregard the Chinese demonstration. The "laboratory" is too large, the numbers involved too many, the twenty-four years of continuous policy too long. To explain the high level of personal morality as but a result of police state enforcement is unrealistic. There is not that much evidence of intimidation. The possibility of improved public health and emotional stability as a result of prudent public and private conduct deserves thoughtful Western consideration.

Chapter Seventeen

PEKING UNION MEDICAL COLLEGE,
FIFTY YEARS LATER

ALL AMERICAN PHYSICIANS have come to their present legal place in society by a carefully described series of steps. These steps begin in high school, and at that point one begins narrowing his options by his scholastic performance (and, unfortunately, by his family's ability to fund further education). Next he begins pre-medical study in college, and here the competition becomes intense, but these college studies are at a remove from patients and medicine. At the end of three or four years of such college work, again depending upon grades and family resources, the funnel narrows and he is in "medical school" (or he is *not* in medical school and begins a rationalization of why he is not, or shifts his target to osteopathy, dentistry, or pharmacy).

Four years of academic studies in medical school then follow. Much of this work is far removed from patient contact and experience. Finally, seven or eight years after leaving high school, he is awarded, by a university, a professional academic degree: Doctor of Medicine.

His course is not yet run. He must now successfully pass a state licensing examination administered by a division of the civil government, not by the university. Is he now ready for practice? More than 85 percent of the physicians reaching this level *do not* go into practice but take one to four years of special hospital training; the majority take three years. Is the man then an authentic, recognized specialist? No, he then must pass a very difficult examination given by a non-governmental, non-university, civilian certifying group. If successful in this final examination, he is then fully "professionalized," a Doctor of Medicine, with a state license, and a certified specialist.

This is a long, long route with repeated checks and balances for quality control. This system has resulted in the substantial high quality of specialists in the United States. It perhaps has also resulted in a large area of health care for which this kind of professionalization did not produce the appropriate and needed physician.

The Chinese were first introduced to medical specialization as we know it through the substantial influence of the Rockefeller-financed medical school, Peking Union Medical College. This facility was dedicated on September 19, 1921, and it was taken over by the Communist government on January 20, 1951. Although other American universities maintained excellent teaching and care facilities in China, PUMC was the flagship for Western medicine.

When the Rockefeller Foundation set up the Peking Union Medical College, in 1921, it did what seemed to be the right thing to do. PUMC set out to carry through a standard of excellence, of professionalism, second to none, and equal to all international standards. Even at that time there was criticism from the Americans involved, some of whom could not see this degree of elegance as relevant to the massive health problems of China. Nevertheless, the standard was set and held to. From 1921 to 1950, PUMC carried on with this program, and its critics cite the fact that in more than twenty-five years of operation, only slightly more than 300 doctors were produced. Almost 25 percent of these left China. Literally none took his career into the rural areas where the millions of Chinese needed medical help.

Circumstances may cloud one's ability to give credit, and among my friends in China there is a tendency for more criticism than credit. Even the prominent Chinese specialist Lin Ch'iaochih, who was in the PUMC class of 1929 and subsequently at the University of Chicago, has clear impressions, right or wrong, of American bigotry at the institution. In her writings, she has described these almost unconscious attitudes and behavior on the part of the American teachers which served to downgrade the Chinese patient. I found these attitudes painful to hear and read about, and I feel sympathy for the original dreamers who undoubtedly thought that by taking the finest of Western medicine to China, they were truly doing the Christian thing. It is regrettable there is not an appropriate means of balancing the scale and for the Chinese to thank these original American efforts—and say no more. At the same time, the American sponsors need to acknowledge the probable misjudgment of some of their original enthusiasm and of their unconscious "imperialism"—and say no more. Too much good came from PUMC (and Pennsylvania-in-China, Yale-in-China, Harvard-in-China, and so on) to warrant the present Chinese attitude of denial of merit and altruistic intent and, equally, too much ultimate success for the original American sponsoring groups to harbor any feeling except that of satisfaction and mission accomplished.

Attitudes may have been wrong, but the harvest of the effort has been to provide the Chinese with a specialized corps of first-class physicians who are giving their barefoot doctor–traditional doctor system a scientific validity and their hospitals professional staffs equal to any, East or West. The Chinese respond to such a reminder with the observation that the Americans should have offered the scientific direction, not the mixture of religiosity and economic manipulation.

Bertrand Russell described this attitude: "Although the educational work of the Americans in China on the whole is admirable, nothing directed by foreigners can adequately satisfy the needs of the country. . . . Americans . . . always remain missionaries . . . not of Christianity, though often they think that is what they are preaching, but of Americanism. What is Americanism? Clean living, clean thinking, and pep." *

PUMC is not now an honored name in China, but its graduates and faculty still provide the senior leadership. For example, at the airport to greet us in 1971 were Chu Hsien-i, dean of the medical school in Tientsin; Lin Ch'iao-chih, director of obstetrics at the former PUMC hospital; Wu Ying-k'ai, head of the Heart and Chest Institute. In addition, in Peking there is Chao Yi-ch'eng, head of the Neurological Institute; Huang Chia-ssu, head of the Chinese Academy of Medical Sciences; Chu Fu-t'ang, head of the Institute of Pediatrics; Wu Chieh-p'ing, vice-chairman of the

* From John Z. Bowers, *Western Medicine in the Chinese Palace* (New York: Josiah Macy Foundation, 1972), p. 60.

Chinese Academy of Medical Sciences. All are PUMC products. Perhaps it was only in the selection of students that PUMC was skilled, but one takes nothing from modern China if it is pointed out that the founders of PUMC deserve a feeling of some pride in the results of their effort.

The Cultural Revolution was not easy for these leading physicians. Practically all of them were early targets and experienced considerable struggle and criticism. Some, such as Huang Chia-ssu, were taken out of the administrative framework for several years.

It is also interesting to note that the head of the leading medical school of Chiang Kai-shek's China is also a PUMC graduate, Loo Chih-teh. He is head of the National Defense Medical Center in Taiwan.

One small index of the difficulty experienced by the China Medical Board (the Rockefeller Foundation group originally responsible for PUMC) in reorienting their thinking toward today's reality can be seen in the list prepared by them in June, 1972. This list describes the present known addresses of "Peking Union Medical College Alumni in the Free World." The use of the term "free world" is a label identifying "them and us." One notes from the list that sixty-nine of the graduates are not living in China. One of the criticisms expressed to me in Peking was that PUMC prepared doctors for the Western world, not for their world. One-fourth of these sixty-nine are living in Taiwan, and this is another criticism heard today in Peking. The complaint is voiced that the students admitted to PUMC did not represent the people but were from mandarin families. Therefore, when these elite families fled to Taiwan, their doctors fled also. Taiwan, in spite of its heavy hand of political restrictions, is identified by the China Medical Board as part of the "free" world.

When PUMC was dedicated on September 19, 1921, John D. Rockefeller, Jr., said: "Clearly whatever western medical science may have to offer China, it will be of little avail to the Chinese people until it is taken over by them and becomes a part of their national life. . . . Let us then go forward with one accord towards the attainment of this objective, which will make permanent on Chinese soil of the best in scientific medicine that the world can offer." Thirty years later, on April 4, 1951, after the Communist take-over of PMCU, he wrote: "But who are we to say that this may not be the Lord's way of achieving the intent of the founders, although it be a way so wholly different from what has been in our minds."

From my own firsthand observations, PUMC has had influence beyond the founding fathers' dreams on the health care system of the Chinese people. True, the PUMC graduates in China can no longer publicly find pride in their PUMC distinction. Given the stresses of the prevailing political message, they may not do so in foreseeable history. However, the China Medical Board should celebrate the success of what was accomplished. Throughout China, leadership positions are entrusted to PUMC graduates, not because of that distinction but because they are competent people with high standards.

The original physical facility itself is in handsome condition and is the most distinguished hospital in the nation's capital. It is also the base for the Chinese Academy of Medical Sciences and the largest medical library in China. There in that library, I have seen the wonderful collection of Chinese classics, but, equally, in the reading room, three men at one table all reading periodicals, one the *New England Journal of Medicine*, the second the *American Journal of Medicine*, and the third the cancer bulletin from the National Cancer Institute, Bethesda, Maryland. The hospital is a national center for continuing education. The chief of medicine and the chief of obstetrics are PUMC graduates. Before the Cultural Revolution, the head of pediatrics, of ophthalmology, of otorhinolaryngology, and of surgery were also all PUMC graduates. Almost all are still in top responsible positions.

I've also been to the faculty residence compound just east of the hospital. Ranking physicians from all over Peking, many of them PUMC graduates, live there. The grounds are attractive, the buildings well maintained.

What better harvest could those present on September 19, 1921, have dreamed, fifty years later?

Chapter Eighteen

SOME ARE MORE STRESSED
THAN OTHERS
IN A CLASSLESS SOCIETY

༿༿༿༿༿༿

WHAT NEW HEALTH PROBLEMS may be arising as a result of the better standards of living and health? The two areas that are immediately and repeatedly apparent are the risks from excessive smoking and the risk of coronary artery disease. I do not deliberately omit cancer, but it does not seem to be a *new* risk. Cancer undoubtedly will affect more people now that more people are surviving to middle and old age; however, I am not certain that there is evidence of increased incidence of cancer. Cancer of the liver and esophagus have always been common; these are two frequent sites for cancer in the Chinese.

Is there any new epidemic which the Chinese people and thus Chinese medicine must now face? From repeated visits to hospitals throughout China, from in-depth consultations on cardiovascular cases at all levels of Chinese society, from data presented to me by medical staffs in Shanghai, Peking, Sian, Wuhan, Changsha, and Canton, I became aware of the considerable and increasing prevalence of angina pectoris, myocardial infarction, stroke, and hypertension. I identify these with no sense of discovery; the Chinese physicians are well aware of these almost suddenly exacerbated problems.

The explanation lies in part in the fact that more Chinese are living into atherosclerotic years, and, not to be forgotten, the wide availability of medical care, which makes recognition of disease possible.

However, I am impressed by the frequency of these problems in the *middle management structure* of new China. All of the accomplishments of these past twenty years attributed to Mao Tse-tung had to be carried through by the loyal, committed Party members and cadres. It is this group of people, as well as the managers in industry, in the communes, in the military, in the bureaus, which has carried the actual day-to-day responsibility for results. This is the group where tension and stress come to rest. Even in a communistic country, all people are not equal, some are more stressed than others. Success and the implementation of the central Party directives hinged (and hinge) upon the ability of the cadre to persuade and, in a real sense, to deliver. Progress upward in the Party, or downward, is a realistic issue.

Combining high responsibility with relatively little policy authority generates tension. The non-mobile nature of the Chinese society makes it difficult to shrug off problems by asking for a transfer or, as one does in the United States, moving to California.

The basic stress-provoking situations have very often been combined in these same individuals with a marked decrease in physical activity, compared to their years in the fields or in the army. This lack of physical fitness is coincident with two of the fringe benefits of the management job. The cadre now has considerably more food, and because of the press of his work, very often is driven by automobile. His own muscle power is no longer needed.

Many of these men have come all the way with the Communist Party and army from the days before liberation (1949), when they were the young, tough fiber of Mao's revolutionary government. Back then, they were the young Red Devils, serving as aides, orderlies, and understudies. Now they are in their forties and fifties and, although not soft in spirit or commitment, they have been physically softened by the fringe pressures and benefits of management.

Almost as a trademark of their dedication, they have been enthusiastic cigarette smokers. The proscriptions of Communist living rule out essentially all of the evident paraphernalia of pleasure. Gambling, high living, extracurricular women, clothes, jewels, furniture, paintings, travel, fancy home are all taboo.

One's options are to be a prime example of a classless society or face Struggle—Criticism—Transformation. As Reston said, perhaps quoting Snow, "Modern China is a sinkhole of morality."

The cadres are the direct arm for carrying out the defined policy of the Central Committee. The one obviously endorsed form of personal indulgence is cigarette smoking. When all else is off limits, cigarettes perhaps offer not only solace but evidence of team membership. At every point, factory, hospital, commune, meal . . . in any possible circumstance, cigarettes are offered, and walnut-stained fingers, all the way down to the second joint, pluck a cigarette, flame it with a lighter, and inhale thoroughly and completely. The burned-out cigarette stub is one-half to one inch long. One, two, and three packs a day are a standard practice.

In the United States, the effect of tobacco on the heart and lungs is not a completely told story; however, the personal behavior of three groups of American medical specialists is probably more important than absolute data. Among heart specialists, one just does not see cigarettes. The same is true with lung specialists and radiologists. The latter group has developed its caution because of the repeated reminder of disease as seen on chest X-rays and in relationship to cigarettes.

The Chinese, including the medical profession, are not impressed by this evidence, and not only does the general population smoke, but, with enthusiasm, so do the doctors.

As with many characteristics of life in Today's China, it is not simple to appraise this enthusiasm for smoking. One wonders how much of the continued endorsement of smoking by the medical profession has to do with the recognition of the liability to one's career if a medical person came out with a bold criticism of cigarettes. One can only suggest with sympathy that the better part of judgment on the part of the medical profession is to put their energy into Party endorsed efforts—and not take on the lonely, hazardous route of criticizing the Chairman's personal habits.

All of the above factors, however, have brought a large health problem into this special stratum of Chinese society. Plenty of food, too little exercise, automobiles, prolonged stress, middle management responsibility, and cigarettes are combining to produce a new epidemic in the critical bureaucracy of China. This problem present itself in several ways, but all affect the cardiovascular system; angina, infarction, hypertension, stroke. As the Chinese settle down into their new network of health facilities and appropriately begin to enjoy their new level of health, which has solved the awful problems of starvation, pestilence, epidemics, and venereal disease, they are very quickly finding their forty- and fifty-year-old leadership struck by this new epidemic, atherosclerosis. Traditionally, we have spoken of "the white man's burden" in another sense. Perhaps the Chinese will need to think of this new problem as "the white man's burden."

In repeated circumstances, I have been able to examine these men, in a variety of hospitals, and have found their middle thickened with fat, their fingers stained with nicotine, and their diastolic pressure slightly elevated. Their symptoms, physical condition, and electrocardiograms are not hidden in a foreign language but are readily translatable into the international language of medicine. Angina and infarction are very common. In one study made of a neighborhood in Peking, hypertension was present in more than half of those reviewed.

Will the Chinese do anything about this new epidemic? One suspects that at the right time and when sufficient Central Committee interest is generated, their national mass line program will thunder out. Instead of "Swat That Fly," one will hear the earnest exhortations, "Stomp That Cigarette," "Cut Down Calories," "Back to the Bicycle."

I give the wrong impression if I suggest that the Chinese, including the middle-level leaders, are not well committed to physical fitness. One of the mass line urgings, over the years, has been for personal participation in "Chairman Mao's patriotic physical fitness program." This is not an idle, unheard message. In Shanghai, at dawn, the parks fill up with solo and group exercise. In the morning mist, the slow, studied movements of the older citizens have a wraithlike effect, unreal, different—oriental. In the streets, hotel and office employees form drill platoons and seem to enjoy a thirty-minute, fast-moving disciplined effort. In courtyards, radios deliver peppy 1-2-3-4 music and plain old-fashioned setting-up exercises go on. All of this is before 8:00 A.M., when suddenly it all stops and the day's work begins.

In Sian, our room looked out on a very large collection of athletic fields, with basketball courts, a quarter-mile track, and soccer fields. From daylight on, individuals and groups covered the entire area. On the edges, housewives and elderly men would set their own pace and quietly, serenely begin their day with their version of Patriotic Physical Fitness. Some would work together, with staves, and go through a duellike effort, often with a coach. The entire action did not begin at any one time, but quietly, from the shadows, one by one, the citizens stepped out and went through their period of exercise, and again, without signal, each calmly disappeared from the field.

In Chang-sha, a large gathering of army personnel was in our hotel for a several-day meeting. There are no rank insignia, but from their ages one could assume there was a general or two, and on down to majors. In the hotel, there was a Chinese-American faculty member from Yale, a small party of young Japanese, and our party of four. The remainder of the hotel was reserved for the military meeting. This use of large hotels to gather cadres, officers, women and youth leaders, and so on, we noted throughout China. The Central Committee may define the policy, but at the province level there are constant management gatherings in the major hotels. In the American sense, these are very similar to company conventions, whereby the company's message and product are dinned into the sales management. Mao Tse-tung Thought is the sales message in China, and the hotels are almost fully occupied by this activity. Many Americans, hoping for visas to China, need to be aware of this prior commitment on hotel and travel space. The Chinese are very busy using their own resources themselves.

Each morning, the army officers at the hotel went through a jogging-in-formation exercise, counting out the cadence, for thirty minutes. This was not token effort but was a realistic "run and sweat" performance. This undoubtedly burned a few calories, tightened a few muscles, and quickened the circulation. I could not help noting, however, the almost constant tendency toward being overweight, exactly like their American counterparts. No one was gross, but the twenty-pound middle padding was there.

The fight to keep down weight must be burdened by the unusually satisfying quality of Chinese food. I won't comment about the pleasure of Chinese eating, but it is certainly one of the first expectations to come to mind as I plan each trip to China.

Finally, as quite a surprise to me, there is the nationwide custom of a two- to three-hour break at noon, practically always including a clothes-off nap. This is a national habit and certainly would not add appreciably to the dissipation of the calories at the noon meal. All visitors to China find themselves urged, at about twelve noon, to "take a little rest." The Chinese do—while the guest rushes out into the street to see the sights and take pictures, and wonders why his host seems more rested when evening comes.

Will traditional medicine have a role to play in countering atherosclerosis and hypertension? This is a question of major interest to the rest of the world. There appears to be no single agent from the "treasure house of traditional medicine" which today can be called a specific treatment for these problems. After all, "high cholesterol" in the blood was an unknown issue in traditional medicine's past. It is a new clue, and its significance is not completely understood in the West or the East. Empirical, trial-and-error testing of herbal remedies will take years of work. Specific projects are under way, however, in the use of traditional concepts in the treatment of heart attacks, cardiogenic shock, angina, and hypertension. Such work will be slow and careful judgment will be used before research reports are allowed to appear in the *Chinese Medical Journal*. The Western- and scientifically trained Chinese physicians and scientists have bowed to the Central Committee's demand for study of traditional medicine, including herbs and acupuncture. This does not mean they will not be critical and accurate. Much of the present research is far too subjective, and accurate scientific standards have not always prevailed. As the Cultural Revolution cools, the very competent, top-quality Chinese investigator will gradually be heard again in the upper circles of the Academy of Medical Sciences, the Chinese Medical Association, the Chinese Academy of Sciences. Caution and concern for uncritical enthusiasm will be their message. On each trip, I have seen the steady movement in this direction and the gradual emergence of the scientific voice of moderation.

For several years, there has been a national drive against acute and chronic bronchitis. Hacking coughing with great throat-clearing noises makes part of the background sounds of China. Spitting on the sidewalk in condemned, and public cuspidors are everywhere. In addition to this more or less chronic "hawking" problem, the Chinese suffer from severe bronchitis attacks, and this illness, in its acute and chronic form, is the target for a considerable health campaign. The problem is aggravated in the north by the steady dusty and gritty winds swirling in from the Gobi Desert. Some cities certainly have visible air pollution from factory exhaust. This pollution is not ignored, and efforts are made to enforce control measures, but there are still problems. Smoke is also generated from the uniform use of open charcoal fires for domestic cooking. Evening time in Peking, as the winds quiet, is also the time when all dwellings, feeding eight million people, begin their open-fire cooking. These irritants—dust, factory exhaust, cooking smoke—are certainly added to by the national use of tobacco. I found it interesting that the national anti-bronchitis drive did not include warnings about the possible irritation from cigarettes.

The Chinese, as do the Japanese, make widespread use of the gauze face mask in efforts to protect the individual from upper respiratory infection. A crowded bus with all passangers masked is not an uncommon sight. Serious epidemiologic studies on the effectiveness of this gauze barrier in intercepting nose and throat organisms is certainly needed. Again, the arena is much more than herbs and acupuncture.

Chapter Nineteen

THE WORLD'S LARGEST
MEDICAL PRACTICE

THE SOCIAL ARRANGEMENT whereby one with a health problem seeks medical help is an understood contract in all societies at all times. Most societies have created a recognized training program and a degree for the medical worker, and in the United States it is understood that the person is a physician, an M.D. or a D.O. When one is sick, big problem or little problem, one goes to his doctor. The arrangement is a personal one, and most Americans can identify a specific physician as "their" doctor. In fact, many Americans have a complete collection of "their" doctors—one for the children, one for the woman of the family, one for their eyes, one for their annual checkup, and so on.

This constellation of physicians has gradually evolved as the American answer to the specialization of the physician, and from this has developed the concept of group practice. A very successful group practice still leaves unanswered the question most of us ask, "Who is *my* doctor?" We all want good care, and in the United States, if one can assemble a collection of dependable physicians who will take care of the various things that can happen to a family, the chances are good of getting absolutely first-class care. If one develops a problem that from the first is straightforward and the specialty need is clear, then the subsequent care will be dependable and good.

If the American has a completely non-specific or even nondescript feeling and seeks care, then the issue becomes more difficult. Or if the family would like to put their confidence in one place, so-called "one stop service," and have one physician who listens, counsels, helps, guides, defends . . . for all the things the family health needs include, then indeed the issue becomes murky.

If one lives on a farm, or is poor, or has a catastrophic medical expense, then our health system's flaws become all too real.

The United States' social system called medicine has not solved these basic missing factors: a uniformly available health care system that all can afford, the personal family physician who takes care of all the first things (the primary things) that can happen to a family; and the physician's helper who is even more readily available and able to do all the things which do not require a doctor's skill. That is not quite true if you live in the right place and have sufficient income; you may come under the care of a dedicated physician and his staff, who will escort you through the medical maze. But for many this does not happen.

Solutions are in motion, and there are those who maintain that the present surge of building new medical schools and enlarging classes will solve this manpower problem. This is not a logical analysis. Although I am heavily involved in the development of one of these new schools, I do not in the least think production of more physicians alone will create here in the United States the *availability* of medical help which is now missing.

Serious efforts are being made to persuade the new physician to direct his training toward learning the skills of family medicine, or, as it is called, primary care medicine. Here again, this effort will not solve the problem. Why?

The reason why neither more physicians nor changing their training will bring a solution to the "shortage" of primary physicians is a mixture of professional, social, and financial issues.

The professional liability in directing one's career into primary care, family care medicine is the overwhelming flood of minor, unchallenging, time-consuming demands which the public places on such committed individuals. The intelligent young person, compassionate as he may be, cannot find sufficient use for his valid skills if he becomes the front line, primary contact health worker. In our society, the financial reward is also missing. To become competent and to be genuinely dependable and safe, the young physician probably needs six to eight years of study and maturation. When he reaches that level of dependable competence, he is not the correct individual to place on the extreme first line of medical contact with the public. To state it differently, a filter system is needed. This system must be wide open at the public end so that any health problem, no matter how small or even how imagined, has access to it. The distance in time or money between this very first contact and the well-prepared physician should be zero. No dollar factor or bureaucracy should come between. The patient must know in full confidence that physician care is readily available if it is needed. However, the endless daily minutiae—shots, cough medicine, school physicals, blood tests, blood pressure, listening, checking, and so on—need to be absorbed by the filter system and thereby preserve the physician for those problems which merit his special level of training.

The initial filter in the United States is just beginning to be developed, and over these next several years, if we do the right things, this role will be filled by several varieties of "physician extenders." Nurses are of course the initial logical answer, and with special training they are an ideal physician associate, as a *nurse-clinician.* Another health professional, already often recognized as a friendly neighborhood medical consultant, is the pharmacist. With but a slight change in their education, these professionals can readily become *clinical pharmacists* and active members of the health care team, not only in the drugstore but in the hospital, clinic, and doctor's office. The combination of the nurse-clinician and the clinical pharmacist, working as members of a professional team with the physician, may be one American solution. The nurse's legality as one who can touch, examine, inject, do, and the pharmacist's legality as one who knows thoroughly about medications, make an almost ideal pairing. Other "extensions" of the physician will be developed from new programs of "physician's assistants," with emphasis on skills similar to those of medical corpsmen in the military.

These several efforts to place another health care member in the American system are all just beginning, and experiments are needed in which a health care cluster of professionals and equipment is persuaded (by monetary persuasion methods) to open outreach health care units serviced by the physician extenders (plus telephones, plus transportation), and connected directly to a more centrally pooled primary physician. The primary physicians would be the readily available assurance of modern medicine.

The United States is moving toward such a solution, but the path is complicated by the territorial preserves of various licensing and accrediting bodies; by the frank dollar issue, wherein the physician hesitates to bring anyone on the team with whom he must share the income; by the nature of insurance policies, which pay bills only if the patient is *in* the hospital (what better way to force unnecessary hospitalization?); by the premium fees paid to the specialist compared to the family physician. Today the heart surgeon can earn several thousand guaranteed dollars before noon, while the primary care physician has worked his way through the mundane but vital problems of ten patients for a morning income of one hundred dollars.

The solution in the United States must tie the urban large hospital to service for some defined area and population about it. This does not necessarily need to be a wedge of geographic pie, whereby a hospital is responsible for a certain part of the city, the adjacent suburb, and the countryside beyond. The mixture of ethnic and religious groups, and the general desire on the part of Americans to have a variety of options, suggest that the best solution in many areas will come when hospitals, with a cluster of physicians, health team associates, and physical facilities, form their own health care packages and encourage families to join them. The contract would include the assurance of neighborhood availability of care and continuity of professional contact, backed up by necessary specialty care at the central hospital at an assured cost. Such plans are happening, and here in the United States some will be called Health Maintenance Organizations. Although some people will think they are a new invention, similar plans have been the basis of the successful Kaiser-Permanente Health Plan, founded during the Second World War in the United States.

Broader thinking will make one aware that I am also describing the Chinese system of health care. The constantly available barefoot doctor is the physician's extension and the patient can move rapidly from that point of entry on to the most complicated of care. The Chinese have arrived at a solution which was made easier, in part, by the absolute absence of a previous system. The solution was also made easier by the Chinese government's ability to define one's social responsibility. If a far western province of China needed medical care, the Chinese, partly through persuasion, were able to move and resettle the necessary professionals.

Here in the United States, the evolution of our hospital-based, suburb-based, specialist-based medical system has produced a highly skilled and expensive piece of a system—but no system. The essential quality of American life which permits freedom of choice and free enterprise has not made changes easy. The professional establishment has not seen readily the flaws in the present physician-oriented approach. Solutions here will evolve, and then suddenly, to the surprise of some, there will be a system. The solution did not evolve in China, and suddenly, to the surprise of some, Chairman Mao had a solution.

The standard of life in China, the rural-based population, and the primitive living conditions of the majority (by our standards) made the problem both simpler and more difficult. The people had no frame of reference to know what to expect; the government essentially had no existing system to build upon. The sequence of events in China, therefore, led to no system that can be readily transplanted to the United States. However, the fact that a system of health care for such numbers of people was brought about deserves our thoughtful appreciation and, where appropriate, consideration of application to the American scene. What can we accomplish by evolution—which in China required revolution?

In China after 1949, vaccination, boiled water, elimination of insects and parasites produced within a decade a new public understanding of health. This was especially true in the rural areas, where plague, pestilence, starvation, flood, war, and serfdom had not allowed the peasant to look up, to see a horizon, to expect more. The Chinese peasant was the original supporter of Communism, he was the soldier in Mao's army; the cadres of today were peasants yesterday. When the peasant began asking for personal medical care, convenient medical care, not just mass line campaigns, then Mao Tse-tung had one of his principal justifications for the Great Proletarian Cultural Revolution. From the beginning of the People's Republic of China, Mao's declared policy, in terms of medicine, had been clearly stated by him. He had called for the admission of peasants' children to the medical school. This had been partially answered by the medical schools, but the failure rate of children from peasant backgrounds had been very high. Essentially, the student body was from urban families of upper-management background. Mao had urged the joining of the teaching of regular medicine with traditional medicine and had made clear his desire that scientifically trained doctors should seriously study herbs and acupuncture and find out what was true and what was useless. Here again, the medical and scientific faculties made motions but paid little attention.

By 1964, the peasant was still obtaining medical care from a Chinese traditional doctor or not at all. If he went to the municipal or provincial hospital, he might be seen by a specialist, but only after a long wait of hours in the clinic, and then given medicines and advice he did not understand. Graduates of medical schools were staying in the cities and becoming specialists in big hospitals. The traditional doctor was not free of criticism. Many of them had no evidence of training, but instead were the custodian of a single family herbal remedy which had been passed down as a closely guarded secret for generations within the family. The traditional doctor would often remain in the larger villages and attend only the more prosperous farmers for an excessive fee. Herbs used in the north of China had different names and different therapeutic claims than the same herbs used in south China.

In the field of medical education and care, therefore, the conflict between the old dreamer of policy, Mao Tse-tung, and the administrative head of the government who had replaced him, Liu Shao-ch'i, was sharply defined. Mao had made the mistake when he reached age sixty-five of removing himself from administration and accepting the role of esteemed leader, free to think and write, but without portfolio. As happens in all cultures, the administration built its loyal management structure, and soon Mao found himself rich with honor, but outside the Party's working structure and no longer able to make the system respond to his wishes. Mao's opening encouragement to the students was, "Bombard the headquarters." The old man, then seventy-three, no longer controlled the cadre system. The very cadres themselves, at the middle and upper Party management level, were followers of Liu Shao-ch'i, and these men and women were essentially interested in stable government, a balanced budget, industrial development, and other forms of logical success in modern government. Mao, in spite of age and personal prestige, felt that what had been accomplished in new China fell far short of the idealism, *his* idealism, with which it all had begun. The peasant had not been brought into the new society as he should; a society of class and status was arising. This was not his definition of Communism. He turned to his primary weapons and mobilized the young to help him. The Chinese youth had been educated in Mao's school system and had been brought up to the level of maturity earnestly believing in practicing Mao's Communism. Now, as they reached out for careers and useful work, they found the doors closed because of "class elitism." With the help of editorial writers, especially in Shanghai, Mao began hammering at his own Party, and, by instigating the Chinese youths, launched his Great Proletarian Cultural Revolution and was able essentially to close down the Party, purge it, and rebuild it.

The actual violence of the entire three-year purge is beyond any measuring stick which we Americans can apply. We have had our inner-city riots, our campus riots, and our congressional hearings, but no event of a similar magnitude, unless one could consider the Civil War as a great national redefinition of values. Ninety percent of the cadres were removed and retrained or replaced. All universities and colleges were closed. All Foreign Office representatives but one were called home. Millions of students literally roamed the nation, physically closing down all organizations and castigating all who did not epitomize the declared ideals of the new China.

Medicine, one of the large social units of any society, was a prime target of the Cultural Revolution. Every medical, pharmacy, dental, and nursing school was closed. All students in school were declared "graduated" and sent to the countryside to practice indefinitely. Faculties were sent away to May 7 Schools and subjected to intense re-education in correct Mao Tse-tung

Thought. The message was summarized in three words, "Serve the people." Perhaps more than any other group, the regular, or Western-trained, doctor felt the hand of coercion. Persuasion had been tried from 1949 to 1966, and the medical teaching institutions and specialty hospitals had misunderstood the message. They had worked hard at preparing scientifically trained doctors. They had developed for new China skilled specialists, and Chinese doctors in their special fields were practicing at international standards. The big special hospitals in the cities were equal to any in the world. By their standard, they had "served the people" and served them well. However, most of the Chinese people were not living in these cities, would not remotely be likely to be served by these special skills, excellent though they might be. China was not cities, and big-city medicine was not useful to a land-tied peasant. Serving the people meant that medical care had to be produced in the countryside—now. Through coercion, through demand, through persuasion and education sessions, programs were initiated at once which kept one-third of the hospital's personnel, from doctor to janitor, in the countryside at any one time. A new health care person was created who was a working peasant with but three months of training as a first-aid worker and the colorful title "barefoot doctor." There are now a million of them in China. He is neither barefoot nor a doctor but is the in-residence neighborhood first-aid man or woman, ready to give care and equally ready to carry out the national health rules. Every city, neighborhood, and factory has similar health workers.

When the medical schools were reopened, medical students were deliberately selected from workers, soldiers, and peasants who had shown their understanding of the message "Serve the people." The children of professionals or of families with "bourgeois" tendencies may go to medical school but will be "specially reviewed for correct line of thought."

With the benefit of a tape recorder and translation, I was able to interview several medical students. Here is a verbatim description of his medical school experience by a student in Shanghai:

"I was born in Fukien Province, my father is a peasant, my mother is a housewife. I enlisted in the army and served for three years, then returned back home and participated in manual labor in my village. I then was recommended by the authority in the People's Commune and by other brotherly peasants to come to the medical school.

"I am very happy living together with my classmates and under the guidance of my dear teachers, and feel I am lucky to be brought up under the Red Flag in New China.

"Our curriculum is three and a half years. Commencing with our entrance, we attended, for three months, a general course in mathematics, chemistry, and physics to review what we had studied in high school.

"Then we went to the countryside with our teachers for six weeks to get in contact with the people and deal with minor illnesses. After returning from the countryside, we again went to the campus and studied basic medical sciences—for example, anatomy, pathology, biochemistry, biology; and we have had a combination course given by the four departments of pathology, anatomy, neurology, and parasitology. We have also had our political study classes, physical education, and military training. I, for example, enjoy running, and I run for a half hour each morning. Our second year, as I understand it, will be entirely in clinical training in the countryside, and our teachers will be our own teachers, but also we will learn from the commune hospital doctors, from the barefoot doctors, and from the county hospital doctors. After that, according to Chairman Mao's teachings—the great article of Chairman Mao on Practice, which says that after a certain period of practice, you must again review theory—we will have further study on certain basic sciences and at the same time we will participate in clinical work in our teaching hospitals. Upon my graduation, I will perhaps return to my commune, but that must be decided by the responsible member."

I recorded similar interviews from three other medical students, all in their first year and all equally New China enthusiasts.

The results of this redirection of medicine are readily apparent in China today. There is truly an availability of health care. It is available where the patient is, and the necessary steps inward or upward to more sophisticated care are functioning effectively. Each level of care seems to be offered by the right level of professional personnel. Highly trained physicians are not consumed by minor problems but concentrate on problems which match their training, and their efforts are extended by the wide network system.

Facts can be tedious but also useful to define a result. The head of the Shensi provincial health department gave me the following data concerning one district, Yenan District, under his supervision. Yenan District is perhaps a useful model to study. It is far removed from the major cities, has had very little Western exposure, is a relatively poor agricultural area with an essentially rural population. Its network of health facilities and personnel is a good working prototype.

The population it serves numbers 1,300,000. There are 2,800 medical personnel, including 1,100 Western-trained physicians (some of them also trained in traditional medicine), 400 traditional physicians, and pharmacists, dentists, nurses, and laboratory technicians. In addition, there are 3,100 neighborhood health workers, including both barefoot doctors and "Red" doctors. The hospital at the highest level is the Yenan District Hospital, and next below it is the Yenan Municipal Hospital. On the next lower level are 14 county hospitals, and at the base of the pyramid 196 commune hospitals (5 of them actually in the suburbs of the city), each containing 10 to 30 beds. Of these commune hospitals, 55 are "central" commune hospitals, which act as referral or collecting points for other commune hospitals.

People in neighborhood districts of the city of Yenan itself go directly to the Municipal Hospital for commune hospital–level care.

The District Hospital is the teaching hospital.

Yenan University has a regular medical school, which has not yet enrolled students following the Cultural Revolution. It was founded in 1959 and had graduated five classes of forty each before the Cultural Revolution.

There is also a middle-grade medical school for the training of adjunct helpers, nurses, technicians, pharmacists, and laboratory technicians. This school has been reopened one year and has 250 students.

I met several "Western" doctors in Yenan District, and three of them had been trained elsewhere (Harbin, Shantung, Kiangsi) and sent to Yenan District to serve, permanently.

One more set of facts, concerning another province, Honan, gives another example of the health personnel distribution. From the responsible member for the health department of Honan, I learned that as of April, 1973, he estimated a population of 34,000,000, and 70,000 health workers ("Western" and traditional doctors, pharmacists, dentists, nurses, laboratory technicians) and 80,000 barefoot doctors, including neighborhood and factory aides.

Acupuncture and herbs, barefoot doctors and traditional doctors, act as the first line and absorb the majority of problems. The readily available backup of regular medicine serves to protect the patient from any dangerous delays at the first stage of care. Regular doctors are being resettled in the commune hospitals, and good second-stage care, including obstetrics, general surgery, simple fractures, general medicine, pediatrics, and dentistry, is handled there. Roving health care teams bring on-job training to the rural area; barefoot doctors and commune doctors have regular required periods in the backup city hospital. None of this health care system is *physically* decorative. The brigade health stations are indeed spare, the commune hospitals are functional, and no more. The *surroundings* of medical care would not satisfy the American. Our expectations have moved us beyond an acceptance of the Chinese system. But if we look beneath the trappings and consider the qualities of *availability, relative cost,* and *effectiveness,* the Chinese have produced a model solution to their problem.

Traditional medicine is very much alive in the cities, too. The public trust in this form of medicine is immense, and one major traditional medicine hospital in Peking saw 1,400,000 outpatients last year. The economic trade-offs of what is not necessarily accurate medical care as rendered by the traditional doctor must be considered. How many people were delayed in receiving care which they should have had? What price tag could be placed on the probable medical mistakes? In this same vein, what price is China paying by turning to a three-year medical school curriculum? Will a generation of doctors be created who have learned to "serve the people" but have little awareness of scientific process? For the short-term gain of getting medical care to the people, will there be a long-range crippling of first-class teaching, first-class research, and first-class specialism? What is the latent hostility and, in fact, fear among the faculties of medicine in the teaching hospitals following the assault of the Cultural Revolution? Regarding this last factor, I can give no answer. I would guess that for many of the older professors and specialists the Cultural Revolution was an experience beyond their worst nightmare. For some, the embarrassment and harassment will perhaps make them permanently shy of commitment and exposure. For most of them, it was a period of readjustment and re-education, but now that they understand what is wanted of them, they are trying their best. This willingness to try perhaps comes from the remarkable nationwide social commitment to serve and also from the realistic fact that there is no reasonable alternative. The latter is a factor, but one cannot become immersed in today's China without an awareness that a historical event in human behavior is being carried off. The successors to the old Yenan revolutionary romantics will undoubtedly have their palace intrigues and violent major jags in policy. However, this traveler's impression is that Mao Tse-tung Thought will continue to be the people's message and that the rest of the world will be influenced by these "moralisms"—if not directly, then by the indirect need to take a second look at their own society's rules.

Chapter Twenty

AN EXPORTABLE SYSTEM
OF MEDICINE

ʷⁱᵗⁱⁱⁱⁱⁱⁱⁱ

THE AMERICAN MISSIONARY medical school did bring Western medicine and public health to China. However, the American concept of lengthy training for a medical professional became a primary area for struggle and criticism in the Cultural Revolution. This "American" concept lost, and has been eliminated from the Chinese social scene. An entirely new approach to training a health care team has been launched by the Chinese. It is not a variant of the Russian, or French, nor any other system. It is Chinese, and if the Chinese are successful, one can only anticipate that many of the developing, so-called third-world countries will follow suit.

The American concept of prolonged special training has dominated much of the world. Many nations have either copied us or their young doctors have elected to come to us. The Doctor of Medicine degree, followed by several years of special training and final certification by a national-level civilian board has become the rule, not only in the United States but in West Germany, the Philippines, Taiwan, Japan, Hong Kong, Singapore, Indonesia, Burma, Ceylon, India, Turkey, South Africa, Mexico, Colombia, Brazil, Chile, Argentina—to name only a few. Many of these countries are poor, and not all of their population has medical care. The painful end result of the American "professionalization" in many of these countries has been to produce intelligent, well-prepared specialists who are not needed by their own country, cannot be afforded by their country, and are useless to the majority of their country's population. This lack of acceptance by their native country means that many of these excellent doctors try to find a new life in the United States.

They are lost to their own country. The United States absorbs these young people as new doctors at a rate equal to the members of Americans being graduated by our own schools.

From a selfish viewpoint, we in the United States benefit, because his native country has fed, clothed, and educated this expensive product up through his M.D. degree. Our country takes him into the system for three years as a lowly paid hospital doctor, and then he finds a place to practice here, becomes a citizen, and returns to his own country only to visit—and see how bad it is in the old country. The United States has indeed benefited, and every community has new physicians from Turkey, India, Thailand, the Philippines, Greece, Brazil, and so on, who are well used here but lost to their own, often desperate, country.

The new Chinese policy has eliminated boards, certificates, and barriers to movement up the health care ladder.

Only very rarely can a student go from middle school (roughly, the tenth grade) on to the university. In fact, I have not seen such an exception but was assured that the system was "not rigid, and an unusually talented student could possibly go from middle school on to further education."

As a general rule, and I suspect a 99.9 percent rule, all students upon finishing middle school simply go to work. This means manual labor in a commune, in a factory, in the army, on the road, on the railroad, or any kind of work which suits the country's present labor need. There the girl or boy settles down and does his job, participates in the life there, and continues his political study.

The obvious therapeutic effect on the American problem of "college dropouts" and "I don't know what I want to do" would be considerable. Equally, the labor pool for cleaning up the countryside, road maintenance, and park maintenance would be impressive.

During this period of serious devotion to his worker's tasks, the young woman or man also tries to demonstrate special enthusiasm as he applies himself to the study of socialistic behavior. The older workers and the cadres watch the youth's development.

Again transferring the concept to the United States, a working corps of youthful laborers would have set times for guided study, for discussions and explanations of the Constitution, the Bill of Rights, the Declaration of Independence, and gain an awareness of what is meant by civil liberties and individual rights. Not a bad idea?

During this period of work and study, the young Chinese can declare an interest in becoming an engineer, a teacher, or, in our case, a doctor. After two, three, or four years of labor, his associates may endorse him as their candidate for medical school. This endorsement specifically certifies that the candidate has shown his sympathy with labor *and* with correct political thought. His or her name is then forwarded through channels. The medical school admission committee has the additional responsibility of weighing the candidate's intellectual ability, but before he gets to that level, he must have the wholehearted endorsement of his local fellow workers.

To jump ahead, the student completes his medical training in three years, and is usually obligated to return to the commune or factory or unit which had initially endorsed him. There is, therefore, a full dispersion of the graduates, not a concentration in the cities. Again, why not apply this in the United States? The obvious and unchanging truth is that we promise our citizens freedom of choice in these major career decisions. The Chinese speak of group democracy, we speak of individual freedom. However, a national service corps with a required two-year term of service after high school, required of all—men and women, poor and rich—would be within our constitutional prerogatives.

Today the Chinese have placed availability of health care above other factors, including international standards. I think they should, given their need. What they are doing may be a more exportable package to developing countries than our very formal, nationwide, professional standards approach. The American society is not commune-based, and it is very mobile, in regard to highways, cars, and population. What works in China cannot readily be tailored to work here. However, just as with traditional medicine, we need an open mind regarding the Chinese innovation in health care systems and health care education. We need to be open-minded for two reasons: first, because there may be ideas we can adopt, and, secondly, we need to be informed about the dominant health care system in the world—one which may become the replacement, in developing countries, for our own product.

In the Chinese system, how do they anticipate creating the next generation of specialists? I place this in the future tense because the new program has not reached that level of activity. The first graduates of this new three-year system are only now appearing. The best description of this new physician is that of a "generalist." I have been advised that the graduate's further training will be by a combination of on-job experience under the supervision of the mobile health care teams coming out from the city hospitals, supplemented by short-term rotations, a few months at a time, in the city hospital. In other words, continuing practice and continuing education are expected to be a part of the individual's entire career. As he reaches new levels of ability, he will gain the endorsement of the senior physicians to do more complicated procedures. A national accrediting body does not have a hand; the decision is made at the regional, provincial level and evidently will be by endorsement of existing trusted specialists in the field. Will this lead to cronyism and ineptness? I was assured that the constant medical practice audit going on at all times would make a senior person indeed cautious about giving a "go ahead" approval to a junior colleague unless there was adequate personal observation of competence.

This absolute blurring of distinction between the various levels of health professionals is a prime goal. For example, a large percentage of the new class at Peking Medical College is made up of former nurses. Their previous training and clinical experience is accepted as valid education, and many of them will be graduated in one year. Furthermore, the new medical school classes of the fall of 1972 had many barefoot doctors in their rolls. Here is an example of a young person with on-job experience plus some formal education who, through demonstration of concern for serving the people, is endorsed by his commune for medical school. One can predict that this will be the source for many of the medical school candidates in the future. This is in reality a work-learn precept and again has merit which seems exportable.

During the years of Russian influence on Chinese medicine, thousands of "middle doctors" with abbreviated training were prepared and sent into the commune and factory hospitals. Here again, "upward mobility" is a basic concept, and through rotations back to the city hospital and visits to the commune hospital of mobile health care teams, many of these men and women have become proficient specialists. At one commune, I met such a middle doctor, now six years in practice, who had all necessary approval for gall bladder surgery and appendix removal, and, to my surprise, was quite at home doing partial stomach resections. Such "middle" doctors, although from abbreviated training programs, are nevertheless "doctors" and do not re-enroll in school for further formal training. This is in contradistinction to the "barefoot" doctor, who is not considered a true health professional but who, if circumstances warrant, may be formally sent to medical school to become a regular doctor.

Wound breakdown, post-surgery infections, and complications are tightly monitored, as is everything in this regimented country. This middle doctor has had four hundred consecutive operations without an infection. His hospital is in the midst of a dusty, fertilized, hog- and duck-filled commune, and one can only admire his ability—and the immune bodies of his patients.

How does one become a "real" specialist, fit for the great city hospitals and medical schools? Here, as in many areas, the Chinese can only say that it is "under study." My best advice, from ranking medical members of the government, is that the same system will be followed, namely, that if a woman or a man has done very well with his obligatory tasks, then his colleagues may recommend him for further highly specialized training, similar to our residency concept. I was told that he will have to have proved himself first, however, politically, professionally, and ethically.

Is there an advantage to being a specialist? The advantages are not particularly in money. The spread of the pay scale is very small. The reward may be in the fringe benefits of city living and recognition. There is no reward to one's children. As they reach middle school, they, too, become a part of the mixed proletariat and contribute at the level that matches their ability and dedication. In fact, one punishment for the city specialist (the elite, as they are called) resulting from the Cultural Revolution is that *his* children must *especially* demonstrate their sympathy for the laborer and farmer. One of my heart specialist friends has two children, both in the countryside at work, one, in fact, in Inner Mongolia. The father can make no effort to reach out and facilitate their return to a university setting. They may return, but apparently must make a major demonstration of commitment. And any leverage applied by their father would be a liability to them.

Will all of this looseness of academic arrangement continue? Will there gradually be a setting of standards and a national definition of rules? One can only suppose so. Societies always formalize and one can only recognize that the personal influence of Mao Tse-tung must pass from the scene. He is now eighty. In his interviews with Snow, he made the frank observation that the new generation will determine the future and that he, Mao, cannot predict, nor does he even want to predict, what will evolve. He also told Snow that he felt that the Cultural Revolution was but one of many recurrent revolutions or shocks which will need to be applied to Chinese society in order for it to move toward his definition of the ideal state. Snow took this message as the title for his posthumous book, *The Continuing Revolution.* An absolute, cataclysmic change in everything relating to medicine resulted from the Cultural Revolution. For the present, a new concept in medical care has been ordered. One suspects that periodic surges of continuing revolution will occur, and, still, formalization of the system will take place. As John Gardner said, "Most systems have been developed for problems which no longer exist."

Such will happen in China; it has already happened in the United States.

Chapter Twenty-one

THREE WESTERN WINDOWS
IN CHINA

〜〜〜〜〜

I HAVE ENJOYED MEETING three Westerners-in-residence in Peking. I think it is correct to call them Westerners, although all of them have long since become Chinese citizens and have identified their lives with China. Rewi Alley, a New Zealander, Ma Hai-teh, an American of Lebanese ancestry, and Hans Müller, German-Swiss, are an exceptionally interesting trio, who, though of Western origin, have committed their entire adult lives to China.

All of them are old friends of Ed Snow's, and of course I met them through Snow's introduction. Just before we left Snow in Nyon on our first trip, he sat me down and prepared a careful map, hand drawn, telling me how to find Rewi Alley's home in Peking. He also gave me cordial letters of introduction to each of the three.

Actually, by chance, I met Ma Hai-teh and Hans Müller in Canton the second night I was in China, forgot to give them the letters, and still have my two Snow-written character references. We did use the map to find the way to Rewi Alley's house, quite unsuccessfully. Snow had very precisely indicated exactly how to walk from the Peking Hotel to Alley's home—except that his arrow ended up at the wrong door. Instead of Alley's he had indicated the national headquarters of the Chinese Communist Party. I have long awaited an inquiry by some "un-American" investigating committee as to why I was seen entering the headquarters of the CCP, Peking, China, at 9:00 P.M. on September 23, 1971. My answer will do me little good—I was really trying to find the home of the world-famous socialist, Rewi Alley, carrying a personal note from the American expatriate, Edgar Snow. Such innocence prepares lambs for lions.

Alley's home is within the large former Italian Embassy compound, not more than a hundred yards from the busiest street in Peking. The walled compound with trees and lawn makes a quiet reservation in the middle of the city of eight million people. Several old Italian buildings are in use, the large Catholic church for storage. On the left and in back of the compound is the former residence of the Italian ambassador, now the headquarters of the Chinese People's Association for Friendship with Foreign Countries, a very handsome building with immense Venetian glass chandeliers and Italian marble fireplaces.

To the right of the entrance into the compound is a two-story house, with full veranda. For years, the downstairs was the residence of Anna Louise Strong, and Rewi Alley had the apartment upstairs. Anna Louise Strong died in 1970, and as Rewi Alley says, with the quiet pragmatism of the ultimately wise, "She is one of the three Westerners buried here in Peking. They are all women. I guess I'll be the first man, if they will let New Zealanders in."

Rewi gives the feeling of one who has lived a very long time, has seen a great deal, and is fully satisfied with the course. A stalwart, independent man, he has now been in China forty-seven years, and is now senior foreigner-in-residence. He has never married. Alley does not weight the conversation with remarks about porcelains, dynasties, or other scholarly trappings. He is simply a complete encyclopedia of folk life in China over the last fifty years. From persistent travel and living in every part of China, Alley has become an overflowing source of large and small glimpses of the China story. The fact that his experiences matched, in time, the history of the Chinese Communists and that he has enjoyed the friendship of the leaders makes a visit with him an occasion when one should listen, not talk.

After Anna Louise Strong's death, Alley moved downstairs into her former apartment, and some of the furnishings are her immense pieces of Chinese furniture. The combination of massive furniture, ceramics, scrolls, and thousands of Alley's books, from floor to ceiling, makes for a most hospitable atmosphere. Alley is now a working author, and all about are the evidences of a working manuscript, notes, marked references. A good book about him is *A Learner in China: A Life of Rewi Alley*, by Willis Ariey, a New Zealander. It was published by the Caxton Press and the Monthly Review Society, Christchurch, New Zealand, in 1970.

Rewi's earlier active years in China were engaged in developing schools, in famine and flood relief, in the organization of industrial cooperatives during the war against Japan. In the last ten years, he has been creative in photography, prose, and poetry. Photography has long been a hobby, and his New Year's greeting cards from Peking carried a cluster of pictures of Chinese children taken by Rewi. Although an old bachelor, Alley experienced the problems of raising children; in his early China days, he ran a boys' school and even adopted several of the boys.

Edgar described Alley in *Journey to the Beginning* as a red-haired, broad-chested, driving man with legs like tree trunks. Alley is now pink-haired, mellow, moves with unshakable calm, and speaks in slow, careful cadence, but he continues to give the impression of a vast, solidly constructed man. He has unusually bright blue eyes and a square, rugged face with a brilliant smile. Always a teetotaler, he enjoys having someone for tea and good talk at about 5:00 P.M. There is so much information about China in Rewi Alley that an entire recording team could be absorbed indefinitely.

My clearest picture of Rewi Alley is one of Rewi and Ma Hai-teh walking arm in arm, very slowly, heads together, chatting away like two upright bears. Both are essentially square in terms of their physique, neither is tall, their strong, stocky bodies of prime manhood have now filled out from cheek to toes, fore and aft. As I saw them walking just ahead of me, I reminded myself that the rest of the world will never hear the really remarkable stories these two Westerners could tell. Although Alley is a professional writer and Ma Hai-teh was described by Snow as "the American who knows the Chinese leaders better than anyone else," the two of them are not interested in such story-telling. In fact, they both are hard at work at their jobs and with their basic dedication of making Mao's China work. Both are unusually trusted non-Chinese, and the degree of trust is made clear by their relatively unscathed passage through the Cultural

Revolution. My relationship with either man is too recent and untested for them to have any reason to bring me into their confidence.

Throughout this book I have slipped back and forth between George Hatem and Ma Hai-teh. This has not been carelessness; he is both men, two men, of two cultures. I have had the unexpected pleasure of a series of visits with Ma Hai-teh which now have moved me along beyond any special excitement one might feel at "how much he must know." Ma Hai-teh, or Hatem, or "Shag," is a pleasure just as a wise, seasoned human being; one doesn't need to ask about the fine print. My first meeting with him in Canton has been followed by a shared trip to the Great Wall, a meeting in Geneva, a picnic at the Summer Palace, a dinner as his guest at the Mongolian Restaurant, two lengthy sessions in my hotel suite with the American cardiologists, a shopping trip, hails and farewells at the airport, and two lovely evenings at his home. He lives north of the Winter Palace on the shore of Hou Lake, just beyond the Ministry of Health. The lake is clear, and he swims almost daily, excluding winter. His immense organizational mass line campaign against venereal disease literally "did him out of a job." Today there is not even a useful role for a venereal disease historian. He has reawakened his earlier skills in the full range of skin problems and is the attending dermatologist at the Fu Wai Hospital. This is not exactly a true statement of his activities, because he is also burdened immensely by playing host to visiting foreign physicians. In this latter task, he is superb and a real asset to the Chinese soft-sell, people's diplomacy. Ma Hai-teh not only is a very intelligent man, but combines this with the wit and guile of old Lebanon and the tough, battle-hardened experience of the Eighth Route Army, and uses these attributes to lead the neophyte gently through the Hegelian use of contradictions and dialectical materialism until—*voilà!*—the recent skeptic finds himself led to an endorsement of all things Mao. I have watched him perform, over a lengthy Chinese dinner, pulling, guiding, rebutting, suggesting, until the eight capitalists around the table were all nodding their heads with enthusiastic endorsement. Incidentally, persistently through the long dinner he sipped from his strange mixture of half orangeade and half beer. I tried it, and it's not a bad combination.

George's wife, Su Fei, is a joy and a bright companion. Their son, Yu-ma, a photographer, is thoroughly Chinese and does not speak English. George Hatem in Peking is Ma Hai-teh, and as a minute reminder of the experience of foreigners through history, upon George Hatem's passing from the scene, his children and grandchildren will have disappeared into the vast Chinese population. The assimilation will be complete in one generation. I thought of this as occasionally, along a busy street, I saw a substantial high-bridged Semitic nose or, among all the shiny black hair, suddenly reddish-brown hair. Little genetic fragments bobbing up in the China sea.

George's home in Peking is a one-story gray house, with several memorable features, the first being the fact that the entire house is involved in admiring the first grandson. Other impressions include the grape arbor over the courtyard with colorful bunches of grapes guarded with paper, so that George can keep them perfect for showing at the festival. Another vignette is George's immense collection of airline liquor bottles, all full, and Su Fei's neat volumes of photographs, going back through the years, some of which make you start. Isn't that a younger Hatem playing ping-pong—with a slender, long-haired Mao? And isn't that Chou standing there with a ping-pong paddle? Some of the pictures taken by Su Fei of similar happy family gatherings are a sharp reminder of their special ties to the Chinese leadership.

Two tasty dishes which I met through George's guidance are the combination of steam bread with a piece of sharp cheese, and a heaping spoonful of coarse brown sugar in a bowl of millet soup.

Both Rewi and George live very comfortable, simple lives. They are happy men, content with how they used their lives. A third Westerner who has also made a full commitment is Dr. Hans Müller, a physician, internist, and now vice-chancelor of Peking Medical College. He is heavily involved every day in a full Party task. For years, he did internal medicine consultations, and when I first arrived in China, in 1971, he was then making the move to his new job. Hans is about fifty-five years old, slender, with dark straight hair and glasses, studious, and Germanic.

In China, one rarely has the privilege of visiting private homes, and I have therefore especially enjoyed the hospitality of Rewi Alley, George Hatem, and Hans Müller. Such living is atypical and rather special.

To get to Dr. Müller's house, one is driven north of the Forbidden City and a short distance beyond the White Pagoda. En route from our hotel, we passed the area in which Mao Tse-tung and other senior members live and noted the beautiful drive-ways and plants, and, of course, the walls and gates.

Hans' house is reached by turning left off the main road between the gray walls of Peking houses and following a narrow, hard-baked dirt road through several windings and finally ending up in front of a typical Peking Chinese one-story house with gray slate roof and gray brick walls. Neighborhood children obviously knew we were coming and were popping in and out of doors peeking at us, smiling, waving, and occasionally clapping their hands. Hans' front door is a brilliant Chinese red, but before I could knock, it was swung open and Hans and his wife stood there to greet us. Immediately behind the door and high wall is an inner courtyard with beautiful blooming plants, potted cacti, and a ten-foot-high stone rock garden. From the outside, there was only the dusty gray brick wall with the brilliant red door, but in the courtyard one noted that the eaves were also bright Chinese red, and meticulous tiny scenes of old China had been painted along the walls beneath the eaves around the entire court-yard. We entered the living room from a terrace on the left, and the floor was white marble, the walls painted clean white, the ceiling ten feet high. All of the furniture was Chinese, and there were magnificent pieces of ancient Chinese pottery handsomely displayed. We were promptly seated on a couch, and Hans asked if we would like a scotch and soda. I blinked at the idea of scotch and soda at noon, and he quickly offered sherry and appeared with a bottle of Bristol Cream. His Japanese wife passed a dish of chocolate-covered peanuts and a dish of cashews. On his desk, just to my right, I saw the most recent issue of *Newsweek*.

I should have added that the moment we entered the house a very large, loud-barking dog rushed around the living room, leaping straight up, in a manner I have never seen, higher than my head, snarling and snapping at me. Hans told me that the dog was only excited and for me not to be worried, that he never bit anyone. The dog's teeth were showing and, as I said, he was snapping and growling, and I must admit I was somewhat intimidated. The dog's name turned out to be Buch, rhyming with "much," not Butch. In spite of Hans being German and his wife Japanese, both disciplined races, they seemed to have no control over this remarkable dog, who cycloned his way about the living room, on occasion placing both his paws on my shoulders as he leered down at me from his last leap. Finally, I put out a sacrificial hand and petted him, and he immediately quieted down, stuck his head beneath the overstuffed chair in which Hans was seated, and went to sleep. Hans told me that the dog was basically insecure and needed affection. The dog had always slept under this chair when he was a puppy, and now that he was too large to get beneath the chair, simply stuck his head under and thought he was completely protected. He always leaped and barked until given some attention.

Their attractive daughter, Mimi, has a spick-and-span room very similar to any young girl's I have seen in a Western home. She was busily playing the piano in her room.

The house is steam heated, and with considerable degree of pride, Hans showed me his boiler. He comes home for lunch every day for the lengthy rest period, as do practically all Chinese. He spends a great deal of his time in the various hospitals affiliated with the Peking Medical School. After a multi-course meal, we sat down in the garden, had a little bit of tea, and exchanged some simple gifts. At 1:30, the driver appeared, Hans and his wife saw us to the car, all the neighborhood children appeared again and with much hand-waving we made our departure.

These three homes are no example of the ordinary Chinese citizen lives, and I tell my story but to draw a picture of these three Westerners and their elected lot in China. All three at one point when young became disenchanted with what they saw, and

the Indian Ocean and to China's freighters. China has health care teams throughout the world helping set up hospitals and clinics and health care systems in developing countries.

China was, last year, the world's largest producer of cotton cloth. China had bought 750,000 bales of U.S. cotton in one year. China has bought one billion dollars' worth of grain from Canada over a ten-year period. China's rice is traded for Ceylon's rubber. The only point in such a recitation is to remind one that the world's largest labor pool, intelligent and skilled, with low demands for personal salary, is about to enter the world's competitive production market. One hundred million industrious Japanese without the benefit of the natural resources needed by an industrial nation, have shown the world but a hint of what eight hundred million "serve the people" Chinese workers, with ample oil, coal, and iron, will generate now that they have, on their own terms, become a major member of the world community.

The ability of the Chinese to work hard has been the prime source of capital which has made possible the gains of the past twenty years. China has used its endless source of labor, and from the muscle of its people has become a modern nation. Snow told me that the Chinese government carefully calculated the man-weeks of labor which were underused or not used, and it was from these figures that national goals were determined. The complete utilization of the entire public's time not only eliminated unemployment and welfare but also was a major factor in eliminating unwanted social behavior such as drugs or gambling. The Chinese simply invested their leisure time in work projects. Leisure was not eliminated—in fact, an eight-hour workday was guaranteed—but, instead, leisure time became time for cooperative projects involving neighborhood and community. These include neighborhood clean-up campaigns, but they also include huge reforestation efforts and a complete underground bomb shelter system. This latter project is surely of a dimension almost equal to the Great Wall, but its reaches can only be guessed. Digging under every city, school, factory, neighborhood throughout all of China represents more miles of tunnel than one can conceive. I was able to see a part of it at the invitation of Dr. Kuo Mo-jo, head of the Chinese Academy of Sciences. During a conversation with him, he made strong statements about the defenses China was developing to protect itself against its enemies, and singled out the Russians and discussed them surprisingly thoroughly. He indicated that all of China's efforts were going into defense and not into offense, and cited the historical fact that the Great Wall was only defensive and that the underground tunnels throughout the city and China were obviously not offensive.

He asked if we had seen the tunnels. I told him no, and he said we were certainly free to do so. I therefore followed through and was taken by car to a shopping center just south of the Drum Tower and there was met by a party of about eight people, in-including two People's Liberation Army soldiers. After much handshaking, we walked about fifty yards south to a very busy department store, approximately across the street from the famous Peking Duck Restaurant. We entered the department store, which was obviously not a plant or prop, since the people there were busily buying and shopping. Approximately ten paces inside the door, we turned between two counters and paused, a young lady pressed a hidden switch high on the wall, and the floor behind the counter slid back into the wall, revealing an opening about five feet by ten feet, with steps five feet wide and fairly steep going down about ten feet. We descended, turned sharply left, and were met there by a party of two, who had padded coats for us and insisted that I put one on. The party started out on a very rapid walk, and I carefully kept aware of my direction. We walked approximately west an eighth of a mile through a complex of clean, adequately lighted, well-ventilated tunnels. These tunnels were about six feet six inches high and five feet wide. They were mortared and bricked on all sides. There were drains in the floor. There was a large six-inch red conduit for bringing in air on the right-hand side at ceiling level. There were two wires strung at ceiling level on the left, and one of these provided the power for lights of the size that we use in our automobile dashboard and tail lights. Military music came from a radio system. As we walked, I did not attempt to stop, but noted very frequent branching tunnels, each with its own iron door, and was told that these led to various businesses and stores, which were connected to the tunnel. We passed a clean restroom with several facilities and a first-aid station, about thirty feet by fifteen feet. We finally turned to our left and then again to our left, and I knew we were circling back to where we had started, there we paused in a room approximately forty feet by thirty feet with a high ceiling.

The room was set up with tables and hot tea and a large chart. We promptly sat down, and an attractive young lady began an explanation of the tunnel system. This entire network of tunnels had been built by the employees and merchants who work in this area, by their own labor in the evenings and on the weekends. The tunnels are eight meters beneath the ground and serve an area of 270 meters by about 100 meters. Specifically, they serve the entire shopping area directly over this network. The young woman stood at my right and used a pointer and traced the map of the basic network. On the east, the network reaches across the main street. Branches lead off to adjacent neighborhood networks, and through these branches individuals can be evacuated to the subway system and eventually transported to the suburbs for evacuation from that city in case of bomb attack. They carefully explained that the network is not entirely finished, but the people in each neighborhood are doing the labor themselves at night. I asked what they meant by this, and they pointed out that 80 percent of the employees of the stores above this tunnel system were women, and they had, on their "volunteer time," dug the network, even fashioning their own digging instruments, and finally had even made their bricks and cement on the ground above. I should have mentioned that as we were walking west through the tunnel system, at about 150 yards we came to a crude but effective elevator system, approximately ten square feet and leading up to the ground, which was used for taking out earth and bringing down bricks and mortar. The employees themselves, with People's Liberation Army guidance, had planned the network to serve their needs. The needs consisted of the ability to bring below approximately eight thousand people within five minutes' warning. This figure is derived from an estimate of the number that might be shopping and working in the area at any given time on a busy day. The food facilities that have been stored are adequate for the employees for several days. The attempt would be made to escort each person through the network to his own region in Peking or to take everyone to the suburbs and out of the city. They feel that their water supply is completely resolved by several deep wells they have dug in the floors of the tunnel; there is a continuous fresh water supply and they have not had to allow for this storage problem.

The meeting room we were in was directly beneath a children's store.

Along the walls of this meeting room were cupboards and counters, which were empty, but I was told that clothing, blankets, and so on, would be distributed from this room in case of a disaster, and that, equally, this big room would be used as the command headquarters. Telephone lines run throughout the tunnel and throughout the city, and there is a self-contained radio system operating from this room. After having tea and an exchange of questions, we left this room and walked west again about thirty paces and came to a very large room running east and west, which was just being finished. This room, whose floor had a black tar seal for waterproofing, was at least sixty to seventy feet long and forty feet wide with a very high ceiling. It was identified as the dining room.

We then entered a final network of tunnels, which were in the process of being excavated and still had earth walls. I had asked during the briefing what the composition of the earth was at this level and had been told it was a sandy clay. I had asked if any artifacts had been found, and they said they had found one deer skull with antlers and had been told by people from the museum that it was probably 500,000 years old.

The tunnel in which we were returning to our point of origin ran parallel to and was the same size as the one in which we had made our original trip west. It was explained to me that the double tunnels had been planned in order to handle traffic and to avoid congestion.

Finally, we came to the easternmost division of the tunnel, and the guide pointed out the door that led to Peking Duck Restaurant. We then took off our padded coats and ascended the steps; the ceiling slipped back, and we stepped into the busy store. Shoppers and clerks paid absolutely no attention to us. Obviously the area was very well known and, also obviously, people have frequently been escorted on the tour I had taken.

I later asked Wu Wei-jan about such tunnels, and he said they were begun in 1969. The call which Mao had put out was, "Dig the tunnels deep, store plenty of grain, and never seek hegemony." Wu indicated that in 1969, 1970, and 1971 a great deal had been done in the tunnels, and he felt that at present the tunneling was essentially complete throughout all of the major cities of China. Wu also said that he thought the building of tunnels had a considerable patriotic purpose in increasing the awareness of the population and in getting them involved in a common project. Wu and I agreed that perhaps the tunnels would never by used but that they had served their purpose in stimulating the consciousness of the Chinese people as to the risk of the Russians. Equally—and this is my own comment—they had given the leaders of China a means of provoking a mass action from the Chinese and getting them involved in a coordinated, purposeful nationwide project that reminded them of their oneness and the value of working together.

Another observation on man and his caves . . . One morning in May, 1973, I was taken thirty miles south and west of Peking to the archeological museum which contains the artifacts found relative to the Peking Man. These were first found in the 1920s, and the museum has been built immediately next door to the caves where they were discovered. This is one of the most primitive ape-human remains which have been found in the world, comparable to those found in Java, in Heidelberg, and in Africa.

We went through the museum and down into the caves and saw where man first learned to use fire and first learned to fashion instruments. That was 500,000 years ago. The caves had been the place in which these ancient ape-humans had taken refuge from the elements and from danger. Five hundred thousand years ago man sought refuge in caves, and now, in May, 1973, man again digs caves for the same purpose. A rather bitter truth.

Chapter Twenty-three

CHINA'S NEW OPEN DOOR
AND THE WORLD

THE REPORTS upon China's state of health made by White, Rosen, Sidel, and myself were unique only in that we were the first American physicians to go, to see, to return, to speak, and to write. In our typical egocentric way, we almost thought we had discovered a new land. Western man has always fostered this attitude and has taken great pride in heralding the seeing by himself of geographic facts as being equal to the creation of them. Balboa is hailed as the first white man to cross Panama and "find" the Pacific Ocean. History books record similar discoveries throughout the world, and "the first white man," "the first European," is the historical landmark by which we have identified the coming into existence of North America, the Grand Canyon, Victoria Falls, and other substantial geography. China's system of medical care is not geographic, but the same attitude, "I now see it, therefore it is," still prevails.

Almost a decade before the visit by the four of us to China, the very competent and respected Canadian neurologist, Wilder Penfield, had inspected China's health care system and had found much which we reported years later, in 1971. He said: "I think I was most impressed by the attitude of those that I met. It was a feeling of enthusiasm, exilaration, and pleasure that at last they were doing something on their own. They were working, especially the younger people, and they were working with a will. . . . I would say in general that there is a feeling of excitement and enthusism among the people." *

Edgar Snow's own observations in the 1960s had been identical to those of Han Suyin, Dick Wilson, K. S. Karol, and others,

* Yale Reports, March 10, 1963.

including respected physicians. These reports, including our own, must be acknowledged as reliable and true unless one holds that we all were led through a carefully programmed maze with scheduled exposures and thus all of us were misled into inaccurate judgments. Such an explanation is impossible when one considers the varieties of experience, by substantial numbers of observers, covering a large spread of institutions and locations in China. Too many people saw too much over too long a period of time.

The skeptic places himself in the hazardous position of rejecting because he does not want to believe the information. Skepticism becomes dangerous when it refuses to recognize adequate data. Accurate information from diverse trustworthy sources about China's health system has now reached such proportions that a persistent critic is no longer demonstrating normal judgment but, instead, the resistance of a mind which deals in fixed ideas. Such minds, which we unfortunately aided in the United States by the bias of government and press, are unprepared and unable to accept the largest reality of our time—that China is now a social and economic force on the world scene. The changes in medicine and health are but a sample of the energy of this social change.

One American who knew the potential of China yet misjudged its direction was John Foster Dulles, who said, "We need to remember that although we have developed more rapidly than Asians in some directions, notably in industrialization, they have preceded us in finding many of the ways to make life richer. Their culture and art long antedate our own, and in many respects have not yet been equalled by our own. . . . They have an exceptional love and appreciation of beauty. They possess in full measure those human qualities which all admire—devotion to family and country, courage and willingness to sacrifice. They possess unusual qualities of patience, reflection, and repose. Therefore, let us not forget that while we have material and technical things to give, they also have things to give. And if we are wise enough to perceive and to take what Asia has to offer, the balance struck between us will not be one-sided by any true measure of values." *

* A report to the nation, March 24, 1956.

Americans living today, and especially those who are young enough to anticipate their prime years in the twenty-first century, are not being prepared for the facts of the world in which they will live if their education does not make them capable of absorbing what is happening in China. This does not mean that one must endorse it or even admire it. However, one limits his and his country's potential if he does not open his mind to every accurate fact about the People's Republic of China. To continue hiding from ourselves what is happening there by the use of mind-clouding labels of "Red China," "Communist China," "Mainland China" is not only bigotry but petulance. The China upon which we placed our bets ended up on Taiwan. It is not the China of the Chinese people. The Chinese people are a whole, intact, cultural mass, living in China, enthusiastically identifying Mao Tse-tung as their leader. This huge mass of people has been united under an operational form of government that has moved their country from civil war and occupation in 1949 to a world force in 1973.

The reason that it is so difficult for us Americans to accept the full reality of modern China is not only our own propaganda of the last twenty-five years but the absence of a historical experience which could prepare us for the modern existence of a vigorous China. China as a great power stopped with the first demands of the West upon China in 1840. From 1840 to 1949, China was never free of attack, economically, theocratically, and militarily. Almost every nation, from small Portugal to massive Russia, and with Japan, France, England, Germany, the United States, Italy, Spain, and the Netherlands joining in, demanded land rights, religious rights, and trade rights. That vast historical presence, ancient Cathay, set off the explorations for trade routes by every Western nation, and caused, almost by chance, the colonization of North, South, and Central America. The very existence of the resultant nations is due to the original excitement provoked in Western Europe by the treasures of the Middle Kingdom. The piecemeal colonization of Africa began because of the vigor of the Portuguese navigators in seeking routes to the silks, jewels, lacquers, and spices of China. The full colonial sweep which covered Africa, India, Indo-China, the Indies, the

Philippines, Formosa, Australia, and New Zealand had its origin in the enthusiasm of Western Europe for finding trade routes to the remarkable Chinese culture and civilization.

Yet, beginning in 1840, the West came close to destroying that which they had sought. As barter for the silks, the English forced opium. To obtain security for their merchants, they demanded the concession of ports. Missionaries came and with evangelical enthusiasm assaulted the Chinese way of life. Resistance to these invasions was logical, yet the West labeled such efforts as rebellion. All of these external forces succeeded in disabling any efforts at a cohesive government and delayed the industrialization of China. China was "discovered" by the West in the fifteenth century with a demand by Portugal for a port at Macao. China tried to withstand the demands of the West through the sixteenth, seventeenth, and eighteenth centuries by closing its doors and living within itself. In the nineteenth century and for the first forty-nine years of the twentieth century, the West refused to accept this attitude as permissible and literally forced China into contact with the rest of the world. This forced exposure brought hardship, disease, war, and poverty to China. Now, united and self-governed, and by a form of government which is alien to the United States, the Chinese people are again intact as a cohesive social instrument.

Not only is China now a cohesive social instrument, but for the first time in its history it is obviously looking out at the rest of the world. China has now opened its *own* doors, and no longer is it an inward-looking society, content to designate all others as barbarian. Instead, new China has a social message and is enthusiastically inviting others to come and experience that message. Equally, new China believes its social message may be of use to other peoples. With the wisdom gained from bitter personal experience, China is not attempting conversion through gunboats. The skilled diplomacy which we are all seeing, and of which we physicians were but a tiny instance, is that of persuasion by demonstration—not by arms or pulpit, but by diplomacy.

New China is abroad in the world, enthusiastic to demonstrate that there is a third alternative in political structure. Just as the early Christians felt they were responding to a "call," so the Chinese feel they have come through their bitter years with a new strength and moral purpose that others may wish to try. The Chinese government has declared itself an ally for all countries interested in revolution. The Chinese are offering their example as a model for the underdeveloped nations.

China will persist in maintaining its own definition of its borders and justifying the rectification of historical losses, such as areas in dispute with India and Russia. These will be word wars essentially, with careful balance between ringing declarations and occasional conflict. China's constant cry of a threatened invasion by Russia may or may not be accurate, but it is a form of Russian roulette which carries risk. Heated charges and counterclaims when armed forces are in daily border contact are a precarious condition. Even if both sides are only blustering for international consumption, a miscalculation or injudicious move could produce sudden, uncontrollable conflict.

The government maintains the entire population in a state of preparedness for invasion, emotionally and defensively. The Chinese are able to see threats on all borders, on the north from Russia, northeast from Japan and South Korea, east from Taiwan and the United States, and south from India. Such a level of anxiety, real or magnified, needs to be appreciated from two views: first, the several centuries of immediate past history when China was indeed continuously invaded, and, second, the utility of such tension in maintaining the entire population in a state of national urgency, willing to work incredibly hard, to accept patriotic dogma, and to suppress their individual ambitions for the national good.

China is intact, under strong central control, but it certainly has not been free of major leadership crises. Mao Tse-tung has remained the symbolic leader, but there have been major periods during which he has lost control of the Party machinery. At the same time, there has been a strong segment of the military forces —army, navy, and air force—which has not agreed with China's hostility toward Russia, or with China's developing relationship with the United States. These elements led to the attempt by Lin Piao to take over the government and call for Russian help, just as had been the sequence in Czechoslovakia. These events also led to the death of Lin Piao. An equally severe policy dispute led to the house confinement of Liu Shao-ch'i, who had displaced Mao Tse-tung as the administrative head of China. For those of us living in other lands, it is important to recognize that these major conflicts at the very highest level did not appreciably alter the historical imperative. That historical imperative is that the largest and oldest culture on earth has survived the invasion of the West and is now enthusiastically ready for the world scene.

I have used the word "enthusiastically," and it is essential to understand the mixture of reasons behind this dedication of the Chinese people. Above all is the full emotional impact of group awareness—that they are the largest continuous culture, that they have mastered and sustained all forms of art, literature, and inventions when most of the world was still a frontier, that their ability to carry out great projects through shared effort, such as the Grand Canal and the Great Wall, equals the feats of any people, that they were victimized by foreign invaders and foreign religions, that the greatest power of them all, the United States, has ignored their existence for twenty-five years—all of these reasons are multiplied by their awareness of what they have accomplished in these twenty-five years. This success they massively credit to the teachings of Mao Tse-tung. Undoubtedly they have had the full effect of indoctrination and constant propaganda. Undoubtedly any one of them who valued personal liberty has had to accept Mao's demand for shared effort and shared reward. Mao has leveled the range of individual privilege, but as Edgar Snow said, "They have been able to move from misery to poverty."

When eight hundred million people have been able to move from vast misery, with starvation, disease, and war all about, and in a twenty-five year period have peace, sufficient food, sufficient clothing, and a disappearance of pestilence and plague, then they are understandably enthusiastic. The six-day work week, the full employment of women, with children in boarding schools from age three on, the immense "volunteer" communal labor in their so-called free time—all of this has not resulted in a sullen, resistant population. Instead, the Western traveler can only report an unusual level of calm, peace, pride, and frank nationalistic enthusiasm. My impression is that much of this enthusiasm is due to patriotism in the ultimate sense of the word, *love of one's fathers*. The Chinese people are again a united, significant nation, aware of their inherited culture and proud of their Chineseness. Communism has been the administrative vehicle and is the official message, but the reason for the peace and pride of today's China is more than Communism.

One can but assume there are those Chinese who thoroughly disagree with Mao's communistic China and its exhortations. The press communiqué of August 29, 1973, following the long-awaited Tenth National Congress of the Communist Party of China, carried in bold print the call of adhere to basic principles: "Practice Marxism, and not revisionism; unite, and don't split; be open and aboveboard, and don't intrigue and conspire. Unite to win still greater victories!" Such urgings certainly suggest a continuing insecurity of the Party.

Continued small peeks into areas not seen by the traveler occur when the world press carries a story that the first and second secretary of the Russian Embassy in Peking (January, 1974) are caught in active underground collusion with a Chinese citizen. And the first-hand report of life in a Chinese prison * sends chills through one's Western bones.

George Eliot's statement, "The strongest principle of growth lies in human choice," may not be adequate to understand the Chinese peasant. Perhaps adequate food comes first.

Is disenchantment widespread and suppressed? I doubt it. The majority of the millions of Chinese have "never had it so good." The twenty-five years of Communism have been twenty-five years of sufficient food and clothing. For the starving millions of the 1930s, the attainments of the past twenty-five years are perhaps well worth the price. The majority *never* had individual liberty. How can one lose that which he never had?

The seeming need for conformity, aided by the intensive indoctrination in school, seems to be fostering personal stability. Will this be at the expense of creativity? How can one know?

* Bao Ruo-wang, *Prisoner of Mao* (New York: Coward, McCann, & Geoghegan, 1973).

The powerful group dynamics now in action has resulted in the world's largest transactional analysis. The confidence radiated by the Chinese can only be described by "You're OK, *we're* OK!," in which the "we" is the Chinese people.

The Communists have moved China into the twentieth century and have successfully pruned the Chinese civilization of the old customs and social rules that had arrested the ability of the Chinese to deal with the industrial revolution. Voltaire, writing two hundred years ago, defined the Chinese dilemma, "It has existed 4,000 years without having undergone any sensible alteration in laws, customs, language, or even its fashion or apparel." Mao and Communism have successfully done the necessary surgery, and the patient, China, is at present adequately grateful for the results and is a willing follower of Mao Tse-tung.

K. S. Karol, a competent reporter, perhaps suspect by many who cannot accept objectivity from a Communist, has compared the two Communisms, Russian and Chinese. His remarks, admittedly biased toward Communism, are perhaps especially useful. Karol said, after his personal inspection of both countries:

"Another factor is that political enthusiasm here is ten times greater than it ever was in Stalin's Russia, and intellectuals accept infinitely greater material sacrifices. Coercion alone cannot explain the frenetic activity of the men who are building China's 'proletarian culture.' These men have not been heaped with honors as were the bards of Stalinism. They do not have private cars, or luxury apartments, or *dachas,* or shops better stocked than the others reserved for them; and they actually go out to work on the land, and afterward they beat their breasts in self-reproach because they are not proletarian enough. They must therefore believe that their efforts will bear fine fruit. Are we perhaps too blasé to understand them? . . .

"But China is a quarter of humanity. She cannot be looked on as a small peripheral social laboratory, easy to ignore or isolate by a new *cordon sanitaire.* The Chinese society of challenge, therefore, worries the great powers, and not because it has expansionist ends; the Americans and the Russians know that China adds up to less, and at the same time more than that. She does not threaten the two great powers militarily, but she brings everything into question because she sets herself up as the model of another form of society." *

One means of trying to understand the scope of the social changes in China is to look at any one major segment which has been fundamental to the new Chinese order and study what has been done. One can look at the school system, the language, farming, or civil functions, such as marriage and burial. These factors have all indeed been altered. The communization of the farms is a well-known change. However, the renaissance of an entire people from abject misery to a level of pride and scrupulous conduct requires the attention of all other societies, far beyond the units of change, such as medicine, or farming, or industry.

What use is another society's morality? Why look to the other side of the earth, to a culture already not understood by us? And even worse, a set of ethics that represents a product of a Marxist mind?

Perhaps there is no useful lesson for Americans to learn from China. In all good faith, perhaps we in the United States must accept crime and poor personal behavior as the price tag for our fundamental principle—individual liberty. Perhaps it is better to maintain the remarkable range of options of our way of life and accept the tragedies as the small penalty. Perhaps this is the right answer. Perhaps the increase in crime is only because there are more of us? Perhaps the raw tide of drugs, odd sex, and pornography will recede? Perhaps the disenchanted young will find, as they season, that the system is better than they thought and take up their duties as citizens?

The rate of spin of our problem increases, however, and even if all the above "perhapses" were true, one then realizes that our system is facing still larger problems. What about the economy, energy, food, excessive arms? Can the same American people with their same Constitution find a sufficient personal discipline to match their personal liberty? The liberty assured to each of us becomes a danger to all of us if we cannot live by an ethical standard that makes liberty worth having. What is civil liberty worth in the middle of a battlefield? And the murder,

* K. S. Karol, *China: The Other Communism*, 2nd ed. (New York: Hill & Wang, 1968), pp. 293, 327.

mayhem, and violence in the United States does simulate a battlefield. Can we learn that individual liberty combined with self-seeking means individual selfishness? We have obtained freedom from many of man's traditional burdens, but is there not missing an agreed-upon and followed moral and ethical framework? Is there not a crisis in our values? Do we not need our own period of substantial "struggle" and in all our organizations—not only the Church—to analyze and concern ourselves with what is virtue, what is our purpose? These are decisions to be made by sensible, not sensual, judgment, not by the psychologists or by the Supreme Court. From the *people* must come an awareness and commitment that life is more than living.

The Constitution and the Bill of Rights are believable documents, well worth trust and commitment. If fully used as guideposts for private and public conduct, then Americans need have no apprehension of the power of Mao Tse-tung Thought. Between the dream and the action falls the shadow—so said T. S. Eliot. And the shadow has been too long and too dark here in the United States.

The People's Republic of China and the United States of America arrive at the latter part of the twentieth century with interesting dilemmas. The United States has devised a method of government, under a Constitution, which has permitted a stable transition of power, through wars and peace, for two hundred years. The degree of individual liberty, the right of personal expression, the freedom of conduct have been remarkable.

The People's Republic of China arrives at this point with an unproved method of controlling and transmitting power. No assurance is yet available for a stable transition. The individual citizen has essentially no personal latitude but must be responsive to group and state. Right of personal movement, of vote, of job, of home, if immigration, has been taken from the individual.

On the other hand, the United States has not developed an effective code of morality and ethics. Crime, drugs, venereal disease, unemployment, racism, school dropouts, broken families, alienated children, alcoholism, graft, political conniving are almost all the highest of any country in the world. The United States has become an old-young country.

The People's Republic of China has been a continuous immense moral campaign, evidently successful in leading the individual into a spirit of patriotism and good citizenship and away from self-seeking. The political leaders have been Spartan, free of corruption (other than ceaseless manipulation for power at the very highest level). The family is intact, marriage stable, children thoughtful and respectful of parents. The Chinese youth is enthusiastic about his government and dedicated to serving the people. China has become a young-old country.

These two systems of living have more in common than at first seems apparent. We Americans have blended our system of government and our religion until it is difficult to separate our country's political behavior from religious connections. Our officials, chosen by the people's vote, confirm their promise of good behavior by a hand on the Bible. We are "one people under God," our expansion westward was our "manifest destiny," with assurance given that it was the Lord's wish. We are baptized, married, and buried by a mixture of civil law and religion. For most of us, belonging to a church is a part of the expected social behavior of a model citizen. Church membership is at an all-time high in the United States, yet a concept of our moral and ethical framework is more elusive than ever. Much of our American credo could be summed up as a belief in hard work, education, sanitation, and God. The Chinese urge work, education, sanitation, and Mao. If one can accept a definition of religion in which the Western supernatural concept of God is substantially that of a moralizer and teacher, then China can be said to have developed the framework of a new religion—the Thought of Mao Tse-tung. The steady transition from identification with Mao as a physical presence to the acceptance of the sanctity of his teaching is well on its way to being accomplished. The development of the phrase "the Thought of Mao Tse-tung" has been the skillful device which gave credibility to the myriad hard tasks demanded by the Central Committee; Chairman Mao's name became the guise for any central command. The codification of Mao's writings, the use of them as the reference point, the gradual transition from the need for his physical presence to the need only for the citation of his Thought, are all part of the establishment of a code of conduct, behavior, discipline, and management. The similarity to all existing religions is a lesson in *déjà vu*.

Two great nations, each with great natural resources, are testing a path of mutual respect and independence. Their mutual needs will force them into a degree of commercial exchange and intercourse. However, the long question of history, not previously presented so clearly, is now to unfold: Is the American concept of democracy, which has now had time to reach its full zenith of power, wealth, and an educated population, a continuingly viable plan? And from the other side, can a full mobilized, regimented, stimulated, Marxist nation maintain its pace, or is the very nature of its system ultimately limiting and destructive?

The export model of our democracy, for which we have tried to make the world safe, has not done well. In the fifty years since the world war fought for that cause, we now have, as our reward, allies and friends living under circumstances very close to dictatorship: South Korea, South Vietnam, the Philippines, Taiwan, Thailand, Greece, Brazil. Our "at home" demonstration model of life under a constitutional, participative democracy is intact and impressive—if one is willing to accept crime, drugs, alcoholism, excesses of personal behavior, manipulation of civil liberty by political parties, patronage, and political favors, all of which may well be the range of latitude expected in such a democracy. For two hundred years the system has withstood variations of such excesses, and still, each four years, the people have voted, expressed their option, and installed a president. The people need equally to consider, study, study together, and instill a moral and ethical framework.

The People's Republic of China has yet to prove it has developed a safe means of succession to power. In the first twenty-four years, there have been successive challenges for the leadership. Mao Tse-tung has weathered all these, and now the blurring of his physical presence into the Thought left behind became the apparent means of transition to his successor. The other unanswered challenge for the Chinese government is to learn if their new "moral" man, who has accepted the rigor and demands of the initial excessive fervor, hard work, and puritanical behavior, can be maintained at this level of commitment. Initial excesses plus initial asceticism are characteristic of successful revolution. How much of the present Chinese model behavior is beyond *normal* human behavior? Mao claims his system is molding a new model citizen. His success thus far is impressive; can such behavior continue?

The citizen there and here can only be appreciative, however, that at least the options are now open for interchange and some influence upon each other. One definition of peace is the absence of war. If only time can be bought so that the large nations of the world can discover their dependence on each other for food and materials, the awareness of the mutuality of dependence upon the earth's resources perhaps will force peace as a permanent condition upon us.

Throughout this book, I have tried to walk the narrow line between reporting what is good and perhaps adaptable by us in today's China and at the same time to make clear my awareness of the precious values which are part of our own system. I refer essentially to those factors of individual freedom which are so much a part of American life that we squander them as a drunk splashes from his tilted glass the very drink he enjoys. The Chinese government has demanded a commitment from the Chinese people which has not permitted room for self-concern, personal latitude, and—what we proudly have—individual self-determination, or liberty. The entire Chinese nation has entered the world political and economic arena as a newly industrializing nation, rich in capital of labor beyond all other nations. Not only is this labor resource able, but it is persuaded that to serve is better than to seek fringe benefits, shorter hours, more pay. Such a national patriotic euphoria perhaps will not last, but for these next several years it is a real and powerful attribute of the Chinese as they begin competing for world markets.

The Chinese also enter the competitive international economic market as very poor people. All other emerging nations can see China as a huge, very poor nation willing to work *beside* the little nations, free of limousines, air conditioning, and servants.

The underdeveloped nations obtain ready friendship from China, encouragement in revolution, ready credit and products, in exchange for their raw materials.

China enters the last quarter of this century as the newest arrival into the industrial revolution, ready and able to see the errors of excessive mechanization and energy dependency. For China, every step toward the year 2000 is one of betterment of its people's standard of living. The United States teeters at the very peak as the world's ultimate example of industrialization and energy consumption. In the United States, one-sixteenth of the world's population shows how remarkably comfortably man can live—if all the earth's resources are available. But the earth's resources to sustain such living are in critically short supply. We Americans have not realized fully that every step forward to the end of this century will require adjustments in our standard of living. One can only hope that in this journey we come to realize that the *standard* of living and the *quality* of life are separable. As one must decline, perhaps the other will rise? Perhaps the unavoidable restrictions on our ability to "have things" and the subsequent increased needs for our commitment and labor will prove therapeutic and aid us in clearing out the errors in behavior and attitude which we all see, admit, discuss, but cannot at present solve.

We have stopped our wars in Asia. Our missionaries have come home. A new missionary, the moralistic Maoist, is about to be heard. The next war will not be with bullets and guns but by the demonstration of the soundness of our respective political and ethical messages and our ability to compete in the international market. Perhaps there will be no losers. Perhaps we will all be wiser.

APPENDICES

THE FOLLOWING FOUR ITEMS are added as an appendix, each to support a major theme of this book.

Appendix A relates to Chapter One and the declaration following the Second Dublin Conference. It was at this conference that I met Edgar Snow, and it was his refusal to sign this declaration that first made me think through the hazards of world peace through enforceable world law.

Appendix B presents two abstracts from the new *Chinese Medical Journal* that has appeared since the Cultural Revolution. These two abstracts elaborate the theme of Chapter Thirteen— namely, that the modern scientifically trained Chinese scientist is looking at traditional herbal and acupuncture lore, and the result is an entire new field of medical science.

Appendix C extends the message of Chapter Fourteen and gives the complete report of the Peking Acupuncture Anesthesia Co-ordinating Group. This is the most thorough article by a Chinese team in the English language. The reader can learn, from this article, the essential message of acupuncture for anesthesia.

Appendix D supports the explanation of how China has eliminated venereal disease, as described in Chapter Fifteen. Dr. Joshua Horn lived and practiced in China and here describes the "mass line" technique of involving the total population in a political campaign—against venereal disease.

APPENDIX A

Declaration of the Second Dublin Conference

DUBLIN, NEW HAMPSHIRE, U.S.A., OCTOBER 5, 1965

The Second Dublin Conference on the essentials of an effective world organization to prevent war declares:

The rights of man and the conditions of life itself on this planet are imperiled by lawlessness among the nations. World anarchy is manifested by the growing frequency of international crises as well as by the number of nations with the capacity to build arsenals of nuclear weapons. One serious adverse effect of that anarchy has been an increasing acceptance of violence and, thereby, a cheapening of the worth of human life.

Protection of the safety and dignity of human beings is generally acknowledged as the highest obligation of governments. The growing inability of nation states to provide this protection, particularly in the face of the nuclear threat, emphasizes the need to replace world anarchy with enforceable world law.

The highest sovereignty on earth resides with the peoples who inhabit the planet. National sovereignty is justified only as it safeguards this basic sovereignty of the peoples themselves. Since, in a nuclear age, national sovereignty alone cannot serve its highest obligation, it must be buttressed by an international authority.

Even if there were no threat of nuclear destruction hovering over the future of the human race, the increasing complexity of international life, the general welfare of mankind and the requirements of orderly growth impose on the nations and on their leaders an imperative to establish world peace and order under an adequate authority.

We therefore affirm the imperative need for a world federation equipped with the powers necessary to enforce world law against international violence and the threat of it. We call upon all heads of governments to move swiftly and persistently for the creation of a world authority capable of maintaining world peace through world law. We call upon people everywhere to recognize the indispensable link between peace, justice and meaningful survival, on the one hand, and the existence of the instrumentalities of world law on the other. And we call upon them, as well, to make known by every means at their command, their insistence that world peace through enforceable world law shall become the first business of their governments.

The Reasons

Peace means more than the temporary absence of major war in an armed world. Genuine peace requires enforceable law, order and justice. In short, peace requires government. In its absence, law, order and justice cannot exist.

The world must be made safe for the diversities of mankind—diversities of race, nationality, religion, forms of government, economic systems and social values. The positive worth of these diversities cannot be preserved without enforceable world law.

History demonstrates the necessity for enforceable law as the prerequisite of order within community, province, state and nation. Experience, reason and common sense compel the conclusion that such law is also the prerequisite for genuine peace on the world level.

Yet it is precisely at the world level that enforceable law is nonexistent. The absence of any system of effective world law precluding international violence makes arms races and recurrent wars inevitable. Failure to correct this basic defect in the organization of human society has now become a threat to civilization itself.

Developments since the Second World War confirm and emphasize the growing need for an effective world federal authority.

Nuclear problems have been compounded by the beginnings of man's conquest of space. Effective world law is requisite: (a) to keep space from becoming a jungle of nuclear weaponry, (b) to head off danger of war from rival nationalist claims to uses of space and planets in it, and (c) to guarantee that scientific achievement in space shall serve the progress of mankind.

Other developments since the Second World War which emphasize the need for such an authority include:

1. The economic disparity between the industrialized and the underdeveloped nations has increased.

2. The break-up of colonial empires has resulted in the creation of a large number of new nations.

3. Five nations have developed nuclear technology and others are at the threshold.

4. The People's Republic of China has emerged as a world power with a population potential of almost a billion human beings by 1980.

The possession of nuclear weapons spreads. World tension does not subside. The arms race continues at an annual cost of $140,000,000,000 (one hundred forty *billion dollars*). With world law, the massive savings from disarmament could be made available to help close the dangerously widening gap between the "have" and "have-not" nations.

The United Nations

The United Nations has helped to stave off major war and has served many social and humanitarian purposes. Through the development of its Charter by interpretation, it has overcome some of its original limitations: It has evolved new peace-keeping methods not foreseen in the Charter. The United Nations has facilitated the liberation of many colonial areas. There have been important declarations of human rights. New impetus has been given to the codification of international law and to new ways of developing such law.

However, the United Nations Charter, drafted before Hiroshima, is inadequate for its avowed purpose. To maintain international peace and security. The United Nations has neither *effective* nor *reliable* means to prevent war. Specifically, the United Nations as presently constituted is deficient in the following respects:

1. Nations having more than one-fourth of the population of the world are not members.

2. The Security Council has often been paralyzed by exercise of the veto.

3. There is no standing peace force to take effective action against aggression.

4. The one-nation-one-vote rule in the General Assembly makes unrealistic the conferring of needed legislative powers on that body.

5. There is no court system with the jurisdiction and powers required for the peaceful settlement of disputes among nations.

6. There is no system to provide sufficient and reliable revenues.

The Essentials of an Effective World Organization

The experience of the United Nations demonstrates that the following elements are essential to an effective organization for the prevention of war:

(1) *Universal and complete disarmament.* The charter must pro-

vide for total national disarmament, not merely for "arms control" or "limitation." This means the *elimination* of all national armaments by every country in the world down to the level of police forces necessary for internal order only. This total disarmament must be subject at all stages to an effective inspection system. The accomplishment of each stage must be carefully verified before proceeding to the next stage.

(2) *An adequate world police force.* Parallel with the disarmament process, a strong, sufficiently armed police force should be established. It should be composed of individual recruits and not of national contingents. There should be safeguards against any undue proportion from any nation or group of nations.

(3) *Universal membership.* Membership should be open to every nation. Citizens of member nations should also be citizens of the world organization. No member nation should be expelled or allowed to withdraw.

(4) *A world legislative body.* The legislative body should be the core of the world organization. It could be either unicameral or bicameral. It should have a system of representation and voting procedures whereby the peoples of all the member nations will be fairly represented. It should be given adequate power to provide for the maintenance and enforcement of world law relevant to the prevention of international war.

(5) *The executive branch.* The executive branch should be chosen by and be responsible to the legislative body and should exercise the authority delegated to it. It must be free from the veto power of any nation.

(6) *Judicial branch.* There should be a court system with the jurisdiction and powers required for the settlement of all disputes among nations and for the enforcement of world law against nations and individuals with respect to conduct which threatens the peace of the world.

(7) *Reliable world revenue.* There should be provision for sufficient and reliable revenues to maintain the institutions and carry out the functions of the world organization. Revenue obligations should be allocated among member nations in accordance with their ability to pay.

(8) *Safeguards.* Important as it is that an effective world organization to prevent international war shall possess powers fully adequate to that purpose, it is equally important that such powers be carefully limited so as to ensure against abuse of power and inter-

ferences with the purely domestic affairs of the member nations. All powers not granted to the world federation should be reserved to the member nations and their peoples. Judicial redress against abuse of the powers of the world authority should be provided.

The world federation should have no power to interfere in any internal revolution or conflict unless the legislative body of the federation declares that such revolution or conflict seriously threatens world peace. The world federation should, in such cases, have the authority to intervene for the purpose of terminating any violence and to bring about a just solution through conciliation, arbitration or adjudication.

(9) *Charter adoption.* The charter of the organization should come into effect only when ratified by a preponderance of all nations and of the peoples of the world.

Every one of these elements is essential to an effective organization for the maintenance of peace.

The prevention of war requires the establishment of an affiliated World Development Authority. It should be adequately financed and staffed in order to mitigate the growing economic disparities between the "have" and "have-not" nations, the continuance of which causes world instability and conflict.

Appropriate steps should also be taken in the interest of eliminating those threats to peace which arise out of discrimination based upon race, creed, color or ancestry.

Ways toward World Order

We believe that the United Nations, through amendment of its Charter, is the best instrumentality for the achievement of the goals we seek. If those goals cannot thus be attained, with reasonable effort and with reasonable promptness, the endeavor to go forward should be pursued resolutely through a supplemental organization or by any other fruitful means.

The time has come for political leaders to put meaning and substance into their generalized statements as to the need for the rule of law in world affairs. Statesmen should now make concrete proposals to bring about world peace through world law.

*   *   *

Edgar Snow would not sign this Dublin Conference Statement. He felt the declaration made too much of the need for world police and peace and did not speak adequately of the need for the wealthy nations to recognize their obligation to help the underdeveloped nations. Snow cautioned against assuming that the Western world's definition of law and courts applied to other major areas of the world. He said that the West's desire for peace was interpreted by much of the world as a desire for status quo, leaving the West with wealth, a high standard of living, power, and the rest of the world locked into peace—and continued poverty—by world law.

E. G. D.

APPENDIX B

Replantation of Severed Limbs and Fingers

RESEARCH LABORATORY FOR REPLANTATION OF SEVERED LIMBS,
SHANGHAI SIXTH PEOPLE'S HOSPITAL, SHANGHAI

The past decade saw a rapid development of the operation, replantation of severed limbs and fingers, in China. Reports of successful replantation came from not only large cities but also small cities and rural areas. Following is a report on the work and study done in this field by the Shanghai Sixth People's Hospital.

Between January, 1963 and December, 1971, 94 cases of replantation of severed limbs were performed at the Shanghai Sixth People's Hospital. Among these, the operation was successful in 79, giving a survival rate of 84%. The ischemic period of the amputated limbs in the 94 cases was: under 6 hours, 43 cases; 6–10 hours, 27 cases; and over 10 hours, 24 cases.

62 of the 94 patients had been followed up for one year and more. Among these, 41 had restored function of the replanted limbs and were capable of resuming their original work; 15 had only partial restoration of function, which necessitated a change of work; and 6 were unable to return to work because of poor functional recovery.

The authors' experience in restoration of lost limbs and the problems encountered in emergency management, anesthesia, debridement, evaluation of the vascular bed, replantation technique, postoperative care and functional rehabilitation are described at some length.

On the basis of their experience in experimental severance and replantation of rabbits' ears, the authors, from January, 1966 to December, 1971, operated on 151 patients for replantation of severed fingers. Among these, 85 were successful—a survival rate of 56.3%. Contraindications to the operation are discussed. Problems regarding bone and joint fixation, tendon repair, anastomosis of digital blood

Chinese Medical Journal, no. 1 (January, 1973), pp. 1–2.

vessels, dilatation of anastomosed small blood vessels, antispasmodic effect of acupuncture on blood vessels, correction of inadequate venous anastomosis and treatment of digital arterial defects are elucidated. Special attention is called to the importance of anticoagulant and antispasmodic therapy in finger replantation.

Through their clinical practice in 245 cases of replantation of severed limbs and fingers and their experimental studies, the authors have acquired a clearer understanding of the primary indications for limb replantation, the causes and management of swelling and vascular spasm of the replanted limb, and the time limit for a successful replantation. They stress that decision to carry out replantation of a severed limb in each case must be based on an overall consideration of the patient's general condition, nature of the trauma, time limit for survival and function of the replanted limb. Factors predisposing to progressive swelling of the replanted limb such as unthorough debridement, the presence of "dead tissue septum," hematoma or infection at the plane of rejoining, anoxia of the replanted limb, faulty body posture, impairment of lymphatic drainage and loss of nervous control of the replanted limb are analysed and discussed. Poor filling, mechanical stimulation, thermal influence, inflammatory irritation and untoward drug effect are all factors found to be responsible for the occurrence of vascular spasm. Appropriate measures of control are suggested.

As shown by the authors' experimental studies, the time limit for survival of a detached limb might be prolonged to a considerable extent without adversely affecting the operative result. The authors replanted with success a dog's limb after it was amputated for as long as 108 hours. Since 1966 they have successfully replanted in 14 patients limbs totally dismembered for over 10 hours (the longest being 36 hours). It is suggested that the time factor should not be considered isolatedly but concurrently with such conditions as environmental temperature, season, and refrigeration facilities. In addition, after the replanted limb has been thoroughly perfused with blood, to obviate edema of the tissues and impairment of microcirculation—both being secondary to degenerative cellular changes in the presence of anoxia—employment of hyperbaric oxygen, human albumin and energy producing substances is necessary.

Observations on Analgesic Effect
of Needling *Chüanliao* Point
in Neurosurgery

Report of 619 Cases

HUA SHAN HOSPITAL OF SHANGHAI
FIRST MEDICAL COLLEGE, SHANGHAI

The results of acupuncture anesthesia in 619 neurosurgical cases are analyzed, with special emphasis on the effect of stimulating point *chüanliao*. If these, 120 were spinal cord operations and 499 were craniotomies. Most patients undergoing craniotomy had tumors of the cerebral hemisphere and tumors in the region of the sella turcica.

The 619 cases were divided into 4 groups according to the distribution of acupuncture points, namely, the *chüanliao* point group (needling at *chüanliao* alone), the *chüanliao* plus body point group (needling at *chüanliao* in addition to points on the body), the body point group (needling at points on the body), and the ear plus body point group (needling at points over the ear and the body).

The results of anesthesia were recorded as excellent, good, fair and unsatisfactory. The overall success rate of surgical anesthesia in the series was 96.3%, with excellent and good results in 65.6%. The rates of excellent, and excellent and good results in the *chüanliao* group (57.4% and 79.6% respectively) were much higher than those in the other groups. Even more significant was the difference in the rate of excellent anesthetic effect in craniotomy with frontal scalp incision between the *chüanliao* group and the ear plus body point group; it was 83.4% in the former and 60.7% in the latter ($X^2 = 5.94$, $p < 0.05$). This seems to indicate that *chüanliao* is the better point for craniotomy with frontal scalp incision. Because point *chüanliao* is located in the region innervated by the maxillary branch of the trigeminal nerve, the supraorbital branch of which innervates the frontal scalp, the better results may be due to its closer relation to the frontal than to the parietal, occipital and temporal regions, which are innervated by the cervical nerves.

Chinese Medical Journal, no. 2 (February, 1973), p. 16.

The effect of acupuncture points located in close proximity to the operative site is far more marked than that of those farther away, e.g., points over the extremities. This shows that the acupuncture points have their relative specificity.

APPENDIX C

Acupuncture Anesthesia:
A Brief Introduction

1. Introductory Remarks

Our country's medical and scientific workers at large under the guidance of Chairman Mao's revolutionary line in health work respond enthusiastically to Chairman Mao's great call "Chinese medicine and pharmacology are a great treasure-house; efforts should be made to explore them and raise them to a higher level." By combining revolutionary zeal with scientific spirit, applying modern scientific knowledge and methods, they have summed up and improved on the experiences of time-honored traditional Chinese medicine in stopping pain and curing ailments with needling. After many years of repeated studies, they have succeeded in creating China's unique anesthetic technic—acupuncture anesthesia.

Over ten years, especially since the Great Proletarian Cultural Revolution, acupuncture anesthesia throughout the country has developed by leaps and bounds. Up to the present time, over four hundred thousand cases have been operated upon under this new form of anesthesia. Implementing the policy of "Let a hundred flowers blossom, let a hundred schools of thought contend," different localities in China have developed many new ways of needling, such as body needling, ear needling, nose needling, head needling, etc. and have done more than 100 kinds of operations successfully in about 90% of the cases.

The successful creation and development of acupuncture anesthesia not only have greatly enriched Chinese medicine and pharmacology, but also have opened up new avenues for the development of anesthesiology. This is another great victory for Chairman Mao's great policy of combining Chinese and Western medicine.

Peking Acupuncture Anesthesia Co-ordinating Group, April, 1972.

2. *Salient Features of Acupuncture Anesthesia*

Acupuncture anesthesia is a new form of surgical anesthesia induced by needling with a special acupuncture needle or needles at certain specific acupuncture points of the human body through manipulation of the acupuncture needles or through electro-acupuncture stimulation producing bodily reactions. The patients under such anesthesia remain mentally clear throughout the entire course of operation; their various bodily sensations and physiological functions remain essentially normal. Only the pain sensation having been so numbed or diminished to such a level that the patients can undergo operations without suffering from pain.

Acupuncture anesthesia is safe and effective. In Peking, more than 30,000 patients have been operated upon under acupuncture anesthesia without a single anesthetic accident. With acupuncture, one does not have to worry about the attendant danger of overdosage of drug anesthesia. Not only it does not interfere with the normal bodily functions, but also it helps to regulate the physiological functions, to fortify the human body to overcome extrinsic trauma; it enables the human organism to achieve an early recovery.

Since acupuncture anesthesia does not require the use of large amounts of drugs, there is no question of any untoward drug reactions. Especially with regard to surgical operations in cases with impairment of liver or kidney functions or in those having drug allergy, the advantage of employing acupuncture anesthesia is even more obvious as illustrated in Case 1.

Case 1 XXX, a mailman was admitted to hospital with severe empyema. His physical condition was extremely weak; cardio-respiratory function was very poor. After several attempts, because general anesthesia produced cardiac failure and local anesthesia could not induce sufficient analgesia, operation had to be abandoned. In 1971 thoracoplasty was performed under acupuncture anesthesia. Throughout the 2½ hour operation, during which 6 ribs were removed and many pus pockets incised and drained, the pulse and blood pressure were within normal limits and the patient talked and laughed at will; in other words, the operation was a complete success. On the same day post-operatively the patient was able to take his meal; three days later he was able to walk about. Recovery was very satisfactory.

Acupuncture anesthesia is suitable for surgical operations of any part of the body such as operations of the head, neck, eyes, ears, nose, throat and the mouth organs including the teeth, tongue, oral cavity and its associated structures, the chest, abdomen, the four limbs, the bones and joints as well as operations in obstetrics, gynecology and pediatrics.

Apart from its general applicability for ordinary cases, acupuncture anesthesia is also safer than drug anesthesia when operating on the seriously ill or debilitated aged patients. Post-operative complications are few and the convalescence is relatively rapid as illustrated in Case 2.

Case 2 XXX, a 70 year old male was admitted to hospital with symptoms and signs of septic shock of 3 days duration. He had a temperature of 41°C, was semi-stuporous and blood pressure had to be maintained with hypertensive drugs. Exploratory laparotomy was performed under acupuncture anesthesia. The gall bladder was removed, the common bile duct was incised and explored and a T shape drainage tube was inserted (30 ml of 1% procaine solution was used during the operation). The operation proceeded smoothly, there were no post-operative complications and the patient recovered rapidly.

In a word, all sorts of patients varying from mild cases to dangerously ill patients in shock and coma, irrespective of their ages varying from children up to 80 years of age, may safely undergo surgical operations under acupuncture anesthesia.

In operations performed under acupuncture anesthesia the patient can cooperate actively with the surgeon.

Under drug anesthesia, the results of certain surgical operations can be judged only some time after the operation. This is particularly true in brain surgery and in surgery of the five head organs (such as the eyes, ears, nose, throat, the teeth as well as the oral cavity and its associated structures). For example, during brain operations under general anesthesia, there is no way of knowing whether or not there is any inadvertent damage done to the sensory, motor and cranial nerves. But during operations under acupuncture anesthesia, apart from the patients' relatively stable clinical condition and clear mental status, through the patients' speech, sensations and movements of the limbs, one can readily tell whether or not the activity of the central and peripheral nervous systems is functioning normally. Thus the occurrence of injury incidental to operations can be avoided.

Also during the eye operation for correction of strabismus, with conventional drug anesthesia, the success or failure of the operative treatment can be appraised only after operation. But with acupuncture anesthesia, the operative results can be seen while the patient is undergoing operation, thus ensuring good operative results at one sitting. There is no question of the patient's suffering from either poor operative results or from unnecessary repeated operations afterwards.

During thyroidectomy under acupuncture anesthesia, the operator and his patient can carry on conversation. This enables the surgeon to avoid injuring the recurrent laryngeal nerve. All these are some of the special and superior features of acupuncture anesthesia. Under drug anesthesia, not infrequently the patient's bodily functions are in a depressed condition. With acupuncture anesthesia, however, the human bodily functions are not under the influence of drugs, therefore it enables the patient not only to resist external injuries but also to increase his bodily resistance against disease. That is why patients operated upon under acupuncture anesthesia recover relatively rapidly.

Because of the fact that acupuncture is simple, easy, economical, and practical, requiring neither expensive anesthetic drugs nor complicated anesthetic equipment, it is especially suitable for medical workers in the rural areas and mountainous regions.

In summing up, acupuncture anesthesia is highly welcomed by the broad masses. It has demonstrated its superior features and shows great promise. Nevertheless, at present there is still some deficiencies. For example, it has not yet been perfected to the level of producing complete abolishment of pain sensation in every case. In some instances or during certain operations, there was either incomplete relaxation of the muscles or the patient could still feel an unpleasant sensation of retraction of the internal organs. These are problems which require further studies for their eventual solution in the future through further practice.

3. Methods of Acupuncture Anesthesia

It generally takes a period of time for people to understand and recognize a new phenomenon before it is generally accepted as such. From ancient times up till now, whether abroad or within China, surgical operations had always required the use of drug anesthesia, so much so that it has indeed become a traditional concept. But now acupuncture can be used as an anesthesia for operation. This is a comparatively new field for many people. Therefore it behoves us to introduce and explain to patients the special features of acupuncture anesthesia, the purpose of this explanation being to let the patients have an adequate knowledge and a correct understanding of acupuncture anesthesia. The mission of any form of anesthesia is to solve the problems of abolishing pain and correcting physiologic disturbances during the course of an operation. Because under acupuncture anesthesia the patient remains mentally clear at all times, only pain sensation being blunted, hence prior to operation one must explain explicitly to the patient all the steps of the surgical operation, and the possible emergence of various unpleasant feelings or sensations. The patient then is fully prepared mentally so that even when a feeling of discomfort emerges during operation, the patient remains calm, being neither nervous nor frightened, thus ensuring the smooth completion of the operation. In addition, in some operations, during a certain stage, the cooperation of the patient is required. For instance, during thoracotomy the patient is asked to perform abdominal breathing so as to overcome the dyspnea incident to open pneumothorax as a result of opening the chest cavity.

PRINCIPLES OF SELECTION OF ACUPUNCTURE POINTS

(1) Selection of acupuncture points according to the *Jing Luo* theory. In traditional Chinese medicine there is a saying: "Wherever the pathways the *Jing Mai* traverses, wherein lies the amenability of treatment." In selecting the point or points for acupuncture anesthesia for operation on different parts of the body, one therefore follows the rule of selecting the acupuncture points in accordance with the pathways of the *jing* which traverse the site of operation. For example, for abdominal operations one may select the acupuncture points of *Pi Jing* and *Shen Jing*.

(2) Selection of acupuncture points according to the theory of "organ picture." Chinese traditional medicine regards the lungs as the regulator of the integument including the skin and hair. Therefore in inducing anesthesia for incision of the skin, one may needle the acupuncture points along Fei Jing (lung pathway).

THE TECHNIC OF ACUPUNCTURE

The hand maneuvre. The needle is held with the thumb, index finger and middle finger, with the fourth finger pressing along side the acupuncture point. The index and middle fingers perform the lift and thrust maneuvre of needle, while the thumb is responsible for the rotatory movements of the needle. Through the close coordinated manipulation of these three fingers, the needling maneuvre is maintained continuously forming a combine lift-thrust-rotation maneuvre.

Why adopt such a maneuvre? This is because single rotation maneuvre of the needle easily leads to the occurrence of a condition called *zhi zhen* meaning stagnant needling. This condition in turn makes the patient experience a painful sensation. If one relies only on the lift-thrust maneuvre, then it is difficult to maintain what is called *de chi*, a condition in which the patient has a tingling, numb, heavy and distended sensation, while the doctor's manipulating hand experiences a tense feeling. Furthermore, the lift-thrust maneuvre alone may easily lead to relaxation of the acupuncture point or bleeding locally. The combination of lift-thrust-rotation maneuvres not only prevents needle stagnancy and maintains *de chi*, but at the same time also prevents the occurrence of hemorrhage.

Depth and direction of acupuncture: The depth of acupuncture needling varies not only with the fatness or thinness of the patient, but also with the individual tolerance to needling as well as the type of surgical operation. For instance, for a fat person with a good tolerance, the puncture may be deep. But for a thin subject or for one with a poor tolerance the puncture may be shallow. Take pneumonectomy for example; it is generally agreed that the needle should penetrate through the entire depth of the acupuncture point whereas in ear-acupuncture anesthesia, the puncture should be shallow. As to the direction of puncture, it is determined in accordance with the requirement of different operations.

The range of lift-thrust maneuvre: It generally varies from 0.5–1.0 cm. If the situation requires strong stimulation, the lift-thrust range should be great. But when the condition requires only a weak stimulation, the lift-thrust range should be small.

The degree of rotation maneuvre: It generally varies from 180°–360°.

Frequency of the acupuncture needling movements: This usually varies between 120 and 150 movements per minute.

Acupuncture needling response: When manipulations of the acupuncture needle have produced in a patient the desired needling response, the patient is said to be in a state of *de chi*, that is to say the patient is so influenced by the effect of the needling that a painless operation can be done under acupuncture anesthesia.

Duration of needling maneuvre: (1) The induction period of acupuncture anesthesia counting from the start of needling up to the commencement of actual operation generally takes 15–20 minutes.

(2) The total duration of needle maneuvering represents the time interval from the beginning to the end of an operation. During this

period it is usually necessary to maintain maneuvring of the needle without interruption. But when the operative procedure causes only small stimulation, the above mentioned maneuvre may be kept up intermittently.

Force used in acupuncture needle maneuvring: This varies with different individuals. For those with a good tolerance to needling or for those in which surgery causes much traumatic stimulation during the course of operation, the force required for acupuncture maneuvre may be relatively strong. On the contrary, those with weak tolerance to needling, or those undergoing surgery in which traumatic stimulation during the course of operation is slight, the force required in the needling maneuvre may be correspondingly weak. Thus, for instance, the force used for maneuvring the needle to produce anesthesia for incision of the skin or muscles may be relatively strong. Whereas while operating upon the internal organs, the force required for maneuvring the needle may be relatively weak. But it does not necessarily mean that in acupuncture anesthesia, the greater the stimulation, the better the results. On one hand, one should judge the results according to the degree of pain supression or analgesia. On the other hand, one should judge according to whether the patient in question feels any discomfort. In other words, owing to individual differences, the amount of stimulation used should vary according to different patients.

On the basis of the application of acupuncture maneuvres, in order to economize on personnel the technic of acupuncture anesthesia by the use of the electro-acupuncture apparatus was developed and is now widely used.

PRECAUTIONS

(1) Do not thrust the acupuncture needle throughout its entire length into the body to avoid fracture of the needle.

(2) When bleeding occurs at the site of puncture or when the needling response or *de chi* is not satisfactory, one may change the site of acupuncture.

(3) After operation, if bleeding, swelling or soreness occurs at the site of acupuncture, treatment with massage and hot compresses would cure the condition within a few days.

CONCERNING ADJUVANT DRUGS

With regard to the use of adjuvant drugs in acupuncture anesthesia, one should assess the situation as a whole. On the basis of having obtained effective acupuncture points and having reached relative analgesia, operations can be smoothly carried out without much discomfort on the part of the patients so adjuvant drugs may be dispensed with. But when upon encountering cases in which acupuncture anesthesia alone is not entirely satisfactory, one may then judiciously utilize proper amounts of certain adjuvant drugs.

(1) Preoperative adjuvants: In as much as patients undergoing operation under acupuncture anesthesia are always awake and conscious, in order to minimize their apprehension during operations, certain patients require the use of sedatives such as dolantin or phenergan to be given intramuscularly prior to skin incision.

(2) Adjuvants during operation: In accordance with the type and extent of operation, whenever necessary, 25–50 mgm of dolantin may be injected intravenously.

When the operative site involves much traumatic stimulation or reaction with obvious discomfort as in the case of separating the periostium or traction of internal organs, one may inject locally 5–15 ml of a 0.5% novocaine solution.

4. Factors Affecting the Efficacy of Acupuncture Anesthesia

SELECTION OF ACUPUNCTURE POINTS AND TECHNIC OF NEEDLING

(1) Select acupuncture points of high efficacy: The so called acupuncture point is a site on the surface of the human body. For acupuncture therapy, the needle must be inserted into a definite acupuncture point in order to obtain comparatively good results. Early in the history of Chinese medicine, it was recorded in *Nei Jing*, earliest extant classical treatise of internal medicine, a statement, meaning that in order to achieve the therapeutic aim of acupuncture, the needle must be properly introduced into the specific acupuncture point.

Needling at any of the acupuncture points is capable of curing diseases; this illustrates "the universality of contradiction." But in order to obtain satisfactory curative results, in a specific disease the acupuncture needles must be inserted into certain definite acupuncture points; this is an example of "the particularity of contradiction." This phenomenon had long been observed by our ancient physicians. Our predecessors through several thousand years of clinical practice had already accumulated abundant experience. For example, such sayings instruct that, for stomach and abdominal diseases the needle should be inserted into the acupuncture point of *zu san li*, whereas for ailments of the back and loins the needle should be inserted into the acupuncture point of *wei zhong*, etc. These time-honored sayings are still applied in daily clinical practice.

Likewise, with regard to acupuncture anesthesia, there have been similar clinical experiences. For instance, in thyroid operations the acupuncture point *ho ku* is most frequently used; in lobectomy the acupuncture point *san yang lo* is found to yield better results. If one does not select the proper acupuncture points, the successful induction of acupuncture anesthesia will be unfavorably influenced. These are the specific manifestations of "the particularity of contradiction." Hence, the success or failure of acupuncture anesthesia hinges much on the selection of the proper acupuncture points.

(2) Need of proper stimulation: Acupuncture can be used to treat diseases, but in order to increase its therapeutic effect the amount of stimulation given should be appropriate. If the strength of stimulation is insufficient, then it will not produce good therapeutic efficacy. During operation under acupuncture anesthesia, usually it is necessary to apply "needle maneuvring" or electro-acupuncture stimulation throughout the course of operation. If the dose of stimulation given is not sufficient, then it would not yield a satisfactory analgesic effect. Does it mean then that the greater the stimulation, the better the analgesic effect? This is not necessarily so. As already stated elsewhere previously, certainly it does not follow that the stronger the stimulation, the higher the efficacy. Because of individual differences, some patients need a stronger stimulation than others, while others need a weaker stimulation. That is to say if one gives the same dose of stimulation to all patients, or if during an operation one increases the stimulation dosage at will, the therapeutic effect of acupuncture anesthesia would not necessarily be good. Concrete problems require concrete analyses. The stimulation dose should therefore be judiciously given according to the tolerance of each patient. Proper or improper gauging of the stimulation dose is one of the factors that influence the efficacy of acupuncture anesthesia.

(3) Induction time of acupuncture anesthesia: Acupuncture can suppress pain, but a certain period must elapse before it produces its analgesic effect. Although in dealing with non-surgical cases, the therapeutic efficacy of acupuncture is often rapid and dramatic, the etiological factors and the clinical conditions in such cases are different from the surgical cases in which the operative trauma is a prominent feature not obtaining in ordinary medical cases. Therefore in giving acupuncture anesthesia, one should bear in mind that an induction interval is required before the surgeon actually starts operating.

(4) The relationship between *de chi* and efficacy of acupuncture

anesthesia: What is *de chi?* This has been explained elsewhere in this paper and will not be reiterated here.

In order to judge whether or not a patient to be operated upon is suitable for acupuncture anesthesia, or to estimate, after start of the needling whether an operation would be satisfactory or not, the main criterion is the assessment of de chi. Generally speaking, if *de chi* is good, the results of acupuncture anesthesia would be comparatively satisfactory. If *de chi* is not good, the results would be less satisfactory or else the case would not be suitable for operation under acupuncture anesthesia. Hence it is clear that *de chi* is an important factor which influences the results of acupuncture anesthesia.

COORDINATION WITH SURGICAL PROCEDURES

The success of an operation under acupuncture anesthesia has much to do with the actual surgical procedures involved, because in acupuncture anesthesia the patient is conscious and mentally clear with essentially normal sensorium. It requires that the surgeon should always strive with the spirit of "constantly perfecting his skill." During the operation, it requires that every surgical procedure should be light, quick, sure, and precise. All these will enhance the efficacy of acupuncture anesthesia.

MENTAL FACTORS AND INDIVIDUAL VARIATIONS

Throughout the course of surgical operations under acupuncture anesthesia, the patients are always conscious and mentally clear. Therefore those patients who have a high tolerance for needling, who have confidence in acupuncture anesthesia, and at same time are quiet and calm during operation, the efficacy of acupuncture anesthesia is usually good. On the contrary, in those patients who are apprehensive and at the same time have a low tolerance for needling, the efficacy of acupuncture anesthesia is poor. In old debilitated patients the results of acupuncture anesthesia for operations are also good.

That is to say, different individuals may exhibit different degrees of efficacy toward acupuncture anesthesia.

5. Preliminary View or Interpretation of Acupuncture

Why is it that acupuncture can be used to induce anesthesia for surgical operations?

As already referred to elsewhere in this paper, there are multiple factors which influence the efficacy of acupuncture anesthesia. But all these are outward manifestations and conditions. The fact that surgical operation can be done under acupuncture anesthesia depends on the intrinsic factors of the human organism.

With regard to the meaning of structures and functions of the different parts of the human body, traditional Chinese medicine has relied on the viewpoint of the unification of opposites for their interpretation. According to this theory, in the human body the contradictions between matter and function mutually enhance one another. Therefore during their normal physiologic activities, they maintain an opposing as well as a unifying action manifested in a state of harmony. The normal physiologic activities between matter and function can only be maintained through the constant preservation of their relatively harmonious relationship. The occurrence of disease is a reflection of the results of disharmony in the relationship of contradictions which are opposed to each other.

The chief role of acupuncture lies in its ability to regulate and maintain the norms of human physiological functions, thus enabling the organism to restore the disturbed equilibrium to a relatively normal state. In fact, such regulating effect is the most important effect of acupuncture. It restores the disrupted functions of the human body to normal. Clinically, we often find that needling corrects both diarrhoea and constipation, and brings a rapid or slow heart rate back to normal. Needling is good for high or low blood pressure, helps those who have fainted or are in a state of shock to regain consciousness, provides sedation for the agitated and helps those suffering from insomnia to get a good sleep. Needling is also efficacious for certain cases of inflammation. Experimental study has shown that needling certain points on the body of a normal person or animal increases the number of white blood corpuscles and intensifies phagocytosis.

We are of the opinion that the effect of needling in preventing and suppressing pain and its regulating effect are interconnected and react on each other, and it is precisely these effects that help increase the patient's endurance to withstand the operative procedure and reduce his sensitivity to pain. Widespread clinical practice has proved that needling points on the body is very effective in stopping pain. Toothaches, headaches, lumbago and pain in the legs, chest and abdomen can be stopped immediately by needling or pressing certain points. Needling also produces conspicuous results in stopping postoperative pain. We experimented on ourselves and other normal persons to measure the amount of pain sensation. From the more than 100,000 observations, we have found that sensitivity to pain on certain parts of the body is dulled by needling certain points, and normal pain sensation is felt again only after a much stronger stimulus than the original is given. This proves that needling the points not only stops but also prevents the feeling of pain.

How is analgesia achieved by the regulatory function of acupuncture? Traditional Chinese medicine maintains: "The regulatory effect of bodily functions or power produced by acupuncture is realized through transmission of the regulatory impulse to the brain via the *Jing Luo*." As a matter of fact what the ancients called *Jing Luo* and what are known today as nerves, blood vessels as well as some of their functions are quite similar. One therefore may think of *Jing Luo* as the regulatory system of the human body. In particular, what is called *de chi* in traditional Chinese medicine is also in agreement with the present day knowledge of neurophysiology. For instance, in normal persons acupuncture produces the *de chi* manifested as a sensation of soreness (or *ching*), numbness, heaviness and distension; here the pain threshold is elevated. But in the paraplegics, acupuncture of the lower extremities does not produce any *de chi* the pain threshold is not elevated. Therefore one should not consider the *Jing Luo* theory and modern physiology and anatomy as being contradictory to one another. On the contrary, one should seriously make real efforts to carry out scientific studies on their interrelationships in order to find out the mechanism of how acupuncture anesthesia works.

From all these observations, it would therefore seem that both the ancient Chinese *Jing Luo* theory and the modern teaching of physiology and anatomy have something in common.

Acupuncture plays the role or has the effect of regulating the human body functions, thus suppressing or abolishing pain sensations. It restores to norms the disturbed physiologic functions and is capable of strengthening the body resistance. Hence it may be assumed that acupuncture regulation of body functions has a material basis. At the same time the patient's subjective dynamic role must not be overlooked because patients undergoing operations under acupuncture anesthesia are entirely conscious; their mental activities remain alert throughout the entire course of the operation. The inhibition of pain sensation is subject to the influence of the mental state of the patient. Although the efficacy of acupuncture anesthesia is not determined by subjective will power, nevertheless mental factors have obvious influence on the changes of physiologic functions.

For instance, patients with mental depression, worries, nervous tension, and fear all can reduce the efficacy of acupuncture anesthesia so far as the suppression of pain is concerned. On the other hand, if the patients have a strong will and great confidence in overcoming their disease, and at the same time possess optimism, are emotionally stable, and actively cooperate with the medical workers, then it would diminish the sensation of discomfort due to operative trauma, thereby increasing the efficacy of acupuncture anesthesia. Hence the role of acupuncture in regulating the functions of the internal organs and the influence of the subjective dynamic role in the regulating mechanism are not contradictory to one another. Here it typifies the dialectic relationship that matter can be transformed into consciousness and consciousness into matter.

In summary, one may have this concept: the regulatory effect of acupuncture on the human body functions is the material basis of acupuncture anesthesia. The selection of effective acupuncture points and the application of an appropriate amount of stimulation are the necessary conditions for obtaining adequate regulatory effects of acupuncture on the functions of the human body. *Jing Luo* is the regulatory system of the human body.

During the course of the regulatory effect of acupuncture, the cerebrum plays the main role. To bring forth the initiative on the part of the patients as well as the medical personnel are positive guarantees for the success of acupuncture anesthesia.

Conclusions

Acupuncture anesthesia has been extensively used in China for more than ten years and several hundred thousand patients have been operated upon successfully under this new form of anesthesia. Nevertheless, in both clinical and theoretical aspects, there are still many problems awaiting solution. In particular, research work concerning the basic scientific principles or mechanisms of acupuncture anesthesia lags far behind the needs of clinical practice. These problems have to be solved as soon as possible in the course of scientific investigation.

The great leader of the Chinese people, Chairman Mao says: "In the fields of the struggle for production and scientific experiment, mankind makes constant progress and nature undergoes constant change; they never remain at the same level." We must strive again and again and continue incessantly with the aim of further developing the technics of acupuncture anesthesia, thereby making a useful contribution to the medical and scientific enterprises in the service of mankind.

APPENDIX D

Mass Line Campaign against Syphilis

To find the millions of cases of latent syphilis gathered throughout the country was an immense undertaking which could not be tackled along orthodox lines. . . .

In a county in Hopei Province, after prolonged discussions between political and medical workers, a form was drawn up asking ten questions, an affirmative answer to any one of which would suggest the possibility of syphilis. These ten questions contained "clues" such as a history of a skin rash, falling hair, genital sore, or exposure to the risk of infection. To draw up the questionnaire was one thing; to persuade tens of thousands of people to fill it in, honestly and conscientiously, was quite another thing. To do this, intensive propaganda and education was carried out by anti-syphilis workers, who were able to make close contact with the people, give them the concept that they should liberate themselves, and enlist them as allies in the struggle. Propaganda posters were put up in the village streets, one-act plays performed in the market place, talks given over the village radio system, and meetings, big and small, held night after night at which the purpose of the questionnaire was explained and the co-operation of the peasants gradually won. . . .

At first in some places the response was slow; few villagers filled in the questionnaire, and some of those who did so concealed one or other of the "clues." More propaganda was done and more meetings were called at which the main speakers were those who had already been diagnosed as having syphilis and had been cured by a few injections. They told of the mental struggles they had gone through before admitting to the clues and of their feelings after they had been cured. . . .

The trickle of diagnosed cases increased until it became a torrent. News of the questionnaire, spread by political workers, attracted

From Dr. Joshua S. Horn, *Away with All Pests* (New York: Monthly Review Press, 1969), pp. 90–93.

peasants from far and wide who came to the treatment centers, eager to be diagnosed and treated. . . .

The campaign went on for two months, covering not only syphilis, but also such diseases as ringworm of the scalp, leprosy, and malaria. Forty-nine thousand cases were examined and treated.

Then the results were checked. Some thirty thousand people who had been "processed" by the trainees on the basis of the questionnaire were given a full clinical and serological examination by qualified doctors. It was found that 90.2% of all sufferers from venereal diseases had been discovered.

The value of the mass line method had been conclusively proved and the baffling problem of finding one case in a hundred or one case in a thousand among five hundred million peasants had been solved. . . . The new approach to syphilis demanded a concept of cure which extended beyond the individual to include the whole community. The criteria for community cure were strict. They included the finding and treatment of all existing cases, a total absence of new cases appearing in the community, disappearance of congenital syphilis in new born babies, and normal pregnancies and pregnancy outcomes in previously treated mothers. When these criteria had been fulfilled and maintained for five years, the community was considered to be cured.

Date Due

MR 8 1995